PRAISE FOR
SELF-CARE IS ESSENTIAL

"In her latest book, Gwen brings her mastery to bear on providing a short list of straightforward, universally relevant, time-tested techniques that puts every reader in the driver's seat on the road to better physical, emotional and spiritual health. It's hard to believe — but true — that something so easy can be so profoundly impactful and transformative. And that is what makes *Self-Care is Essential* a must-read for all!"

— Judy Dimon

"Through simple yet transformative practices, Lawrence guides us towards a path of resilience and self-nourishment, offering strategies and a profound shift in perspective. This book is a testament to her expertise and my unwavering trust in her ability to empower those who give tirelessly, helping them reclaim their inner strength and lead lives filled with compassionate purpose, joy, and mindful presence."

— N. Tamara Ramirez, co-executive director of CODE YOU

"Gwen has a vast knowledge of how the physical body and energetic body are connected. Her expertise in functional movement, anatomy, health and performance make her uniquely positioned to lead and guide you in structures of practice that will empower your life on all levels. She embodies power and brings an ease and simplicity to stepping on the path and meeting you wherever you are at."

— Pamela Fellows, meditation teacher

"Gwen brings an authenticity and integrity to all of her roles, and combined with her substantive knowledge and commitment to those with whom she works, has earned the title of 'expert.'"

— Lisa A. Linsky, partner at McDermott Will & Emery LLP

"As a mental health professional, 'talk' is our primary tool for healing. The tools Gwen provides in this book are user-friendly for all to benefit and have been a gift to me both professionally and personally as a Warrior Mom of a pediatric cancer fighter."

—**Salliann Schippers**, LCSW Behavioral Health Specialist

"Gwen has dedicated her life to learning and practicing physical, mental, emotional and spiritual wellness and it show in the commonsense, simple approach to holistic wellness that she teaches. The practices she teaches are accessible and straightforward enough that they have become a part of my daily routine and changed the way that I approach and meet each day. I can't thank her enough!"

—**Mystie Arnold** RYT, PYFS

"Prioritizing self-care isn't selfish—it's a health and wellness necessity, which Gwen Lawrence illuminates throughout this book. From yoga to massage to goal-setting tips, Gwen's expertise and experience breathe new life into whole-body wellness."

—**Crystal Fenton**, yoga teacher and E-RYT®200 YACEP® author

"For first responders, self-care is a necessity for physical and mental survival. What I have always relied on is exercise, breath work and positive thinking. What Gwen has taught me is exercise needs a mental and spiritual component, not just physical. When you bring that all together, it helps with feeling centered and positive and strong."

—**Jo-Ann Avalone**, retired NYPD 911 first responder

"When it comes to Gwen Lawrence, I could write an entire book. The woman, the mom, the warrior, the survivor, the mentor, the friend, the list goes on and on. Gwen is the most caring, compassionate, and giving yoga instructor I have ever met. Her vast knowledge of the human body and mind/body connection are unmatched! This is why you should trust her and this book for your wellness goals and journey."

—**Trena Zapata**

SELF-CARE
IS ESSENTIAL

A PERSONAL RESILIENCY PROGRAM
FOR HEALTHCARE PROFESSIONALS,
FIRST RESPONDERS & CAREGIVERS

GWEN LAWRENCE

FOREWORD BY LAURA DIMON

PREFACE BY AIMEE DANNAOUI, MSN, RN, NE-BC, CAPA

Hatherleigh Press is committed to preserving and protecting the natural resources of the earth. Environmentally responsible and sustainable practices are embraced within the company's mission statement.

Visit us at www.hatherleighpress.com.

SELF-CARE IS ESSENTIAL

Library of Congress Cataloging-in-Publication Data is available upon request.
ISBN: 978-1-57826-998-3

Cover and Interior Design by Carolyn Kasper
Illustrations by Matthew Sanoian

Printed in the United States
10 9 8 7 6 5 4 3 2 1

MEDICAL DISCLAIMER

This content is for informational and educational purposes only. It is not intended to provide medical advice or to take the place of such advice or treatment from a personal physician. All readers of this content are advised to consult their doctors or qualified health professionals regarding specific health questions. Neither the Author nor the publisher of this content takes responsibility for possible health consequences of anyone reading or following the information in this educational content. All viewers of this content, especially those taking prescription or over-the-counter medications, should consult their physicians before beginning any nutrition, supplement, or lifestyle program.

It is my honor to dedicate this book to the most
essential person I know.
With work
With family
With friendship
I am inspired to know her, grateful to love her
Appreciative of her unending humor
I have had the privilege of experiencing her beauty
On the inside and out
Since we were three years old!
Strong, resilient, radiant, driven, determined, smart...
This book is for you,
Aimee Dannaoui

CONTENTS

FOREWORD
BY LAURA DIMON

When I first met Gwen, what struck me was how she'd defied any cookie-cutter stereotypes. She was entirely unique: lifetimes of ancient wisdom in the shape of a modern woman — a bad-ass, tattooed, Kundalini master, *hot damn* warrior woman — to be exact. Gwen has charted her own course, and her resilience has been tested more than once. In this book, she shares all the tried-and-true methods of self-care that she has seen transform lives.

Over the years that Gwen has worked with me and my family, I've seen firsthand how helping people help themselves — to realize their fullest, most pain-free, and healthy lives — is the engine that drives her. This self-care book is a labor of love, borne out of her genuine desire to help and to heal. I've been lucky enough to have benefitted from her intuitive guidance and healing hands, and I'm delighted to share a dose of Gwen with you.

At age 52, despite being a lifelong, card-carrying member of the *healthiest people ever* club, she was staring down a scary diagnosis and surgery for non-genetic breast cancer. She faced it with as much grace and compassion for herself and others as she could muster. When she emerged cancer-free and overwhelmed with gratitude for the doctors and nurses who cared for her, she began to wonder, "Who cares for the care-givers?" That's Gwen, always thinking about how to use the many tools in her arsenal to pay it forward. After all, she knows that a caregiver is of no use to anybody when her tank is running on empty. This book is chock-full of science-backed, time-tested tips, tricks, and methods for re-charging your battery.

If you feel stuck in a cycle of stagnation or unsure how to take ownership of your health, Gwen's got you. She has spent more than three decades applying and expanding her expertise across all things yoga, nutrition, massage therapy and more. In writing this book, she's culled gems of wisdom across various disciplines, cultures and styles, and distilled a lifetime of learning into the best hacks.

It's safe to say that surviving the pandemic collectively taught us the importance of self-reliance. As a result, the concept of self-care is officially in the zeitgeist, more relevant and prioritized than ever before. Practices such as meditation or aromatherapy — once dismissed as *woo-woo* — have found mainstream acceptance. Hustle culture is out. Burnout is *so* last season. We are stepping into the era of radical self-love, and Gwen's book couldn't have come at a better time.

Gwen practices what she preaches, and doesn't believe wellness has to be overly complicated, expensive or daunting. The wisdom included in the pages that follow will shift your sense of agency, wellness and self-fulfillment. Gwen provides the *how* and *why*, but what you do with those new tools is up to you.

The difference between living a life of ease vs. dis-ease, of nourishment vs. depletion, resilience vs. resentment, is in our hands. With this book, it's at your fingertips. Enjoy.

— Laura Dimon

PREFACE
BY AIMEE DANNAOUI

In a world where the art of caring has become synonymous with sacrifice, Gwen Lawrence offers a beacon of light, illuminating the transformative power of self-care for caregivers navigating the intricate dance of life's responsibilities.

As a seasoned nurse with over three decades of experience, a devoted single mother to two amazing young men, and a caregiver to my mother battling dementia, I have walked the delicate tightrope of balancing professional obligations with personal well-being. The journey has been fraught with challenges, joys, setbacks, and triumphs, but thorough it all, one truth has remained constant: the indispensable role of self-care in sustaining the heart, mind, and soul of the caregiver.

Enter Gwen, a beacon of wisdom and compassion whose expertise in yoga transcends the physical practice, delving deep into the realms of mindfulness, resilience, and holistic well-being. With a compassionate heart and a profound understanding of the unique challenges faced by caregivers, Gwen crafts a transformative narrative that resonates with authenticity, empathy, and actionable insight.

This book is a testament to Gwen's unwavering commitment to empowering caregivers with the tools, techniques, and wisdom needed to cultivate resilience, restore balance, and rejuvenate the spirit. Through a harmonious blend of yogic principles, practical strategies, and heart-felt anecdotes, she illuminates the path to self-discovery, healing and transformation.

What sets this book apart is Gwen's unique ability to bridge the gap between ancient wisdom and modern-day caregiving. Drawing upon years of experience as a yoga instructor and a deep understanding of the caregiving landscape, she offers a holistic approach to self-care that empowers caregivers to reclaim health, happiness, and a sense of purpose.

As I reflect upon my own journey as a nurse, single mother, and caregiver, I am profoundly moved by the impact of Gwen's teaching on my personal and professional life. Her compassionate guidance, practical wisdom, and unwavering support have been a source of inspiration, resilience, and hope, reminding me of the transformative power of self-care in nurturing the caregiver's soul.

In conclusion, *Self-Care is Essential* is more than a guide — it is a heartfelt tribute to the unsung heroes among us, the caregivers who devote their lives to serving others. I wholeheartedly endorse Gwen's work and encourage readers to embrace her wisdom, knowing that self-care is not an indulgence but a sacred responsibility — one that empowers us to care for ourselves so that we may continue to care for others.

With deepest admiration and gratitude,

—Aimee Dannaoui, MSN, RN, NE-BC, CAPA

INTRODUCTION

At age 52, I found myself walking around in a hospital gown, hair net and booties. I was arm-in-arm with Aimee, my best friend since the age of three and the Nurse Leader at Memorial Sloane Kettering in New York City. What was I doing there? That's what *I* wanted to know.

Why was a lifelong vegetarian, someone committed to clean living, daily exercise, a certified yogi, on her way to receive non-genetic breast cancer surgery?

I was angry, baffled, determined to change even more in my life. I was questioning everything in my life up to that point, wondering how the good choices I'd made had led to such an outcome. (Thankfully, the surgery went smoothly and the prognosis was good.)

But while I was in the hospital, I made an incredible discovery. Both during the surgery and afterwards while in recovery, struggling with the side effects of every pain medication imaginable...my nurses *rocked*. These were strangers, yet showed so much compassion to me — a person they never laid eyes on before. These were attentive, strong, beautiful people who gave everything of themselves for me.

It was humbling, to say the least. So, once I was feeling more myself again, I had a thought: who cares for the nurses? This thought touched off an avalanche of thinking about all the types of jobs that entail a commitment to care, providing aid and consideration to just about every human whether they chose to or not, and about how I could help them lead healthier lives.

PORTRAIT OF A CAREGIVER

You are a caregiver, overwhelmed by your work yet dedicated to helping others most of the time...whether you like it or not. Your patient/client load is above the standard expectation, you have a meeting in ten minutes, you still have to finish your reports and scheduling, your calendar is completely overloaded, you have an ailing parent at home. How can you possibly fit all of this into your life, all while prioritizing someone else's needs?

And so you work overtime until your body aches and your eyes are strained. You cancel your workout, your yoga lesson, your massage appointment. You start skipping meals here and there, which inevitably slows you down even more. Your prevailing hope is to be able to drive home without falling asleep behind the wheel.

Most of us do not think twice about putting care routines for ourselves on hold or permanently removing them from our lives. It takes something happening in our own life — a heart attack, panic attack, high anxiety or even worse — before we decide enough is enough, that, "It's time to take care of myself so I can be better and more effective to others." There's a story I've always loved which helps put into context the value of a minute in time.

Imagine there is a bank that credits your account each morning with $86,400. It carries over no balance from day to day. Every evening deletes whatever part of the balance you failed to use during the day. What would you do?

Draw out every cent, of course!

Each of us has such a bank. Its name is TIME. Every morning, your account is credited with 86,400 seconds. Every night is written off as lost whatever portion of this time you have failed to invest to good purpose. No balance is carried over; no over-draft allowed.

If you fail to use the day's deposits, the loss is yours — there is no going back. You must live in the present on today's deposits. Invest it so as to get from it the utmost in health, happiness, and success! The clock is running. Make the most of today!

To realize the value of **ONE YEAR,** ask a student who failed a grade.

To realize the value of **ONE MONTH,** ask a mother who gave birth to a premature baby.

To realize the value of **ONE WEEK,** ask the editor of a weekly newspaper.

To realize the value of **ONE HOUR,** ask the lovers who are waiting to meet.

To realize the value of **ONE MINUTE,** ask a person who missed the train.

To realize the value of **ONE SECOND,** ask a person who just avoided an accident.

To realize the value of **ONE MILLISECOND,** ask the person who won a medal in the Olympics.

Treasure every moment that you have! And treasure it more because you shared it with someone special, special enough to spend your time. And remember that time waits for no one.

—Author Unknown

WHY THIS BOOK, WHY NOW?

I have carefully laid out techniques in this book to cater specifically to the needs of essential workers. In doing so, I hope to (gently) remind you of all the aspects of your life that are slung down the ladder of importance and want to help you remember why they are important to you as essential workers. You certainly have chosen your career path for a reason—and it may well be the most unselfish, noble career there is—but I still need you to remember why you chose this path.

And now...flip the script. Whatever reason it was that convinced you all people deserve help, remember that you are no less deserving than they are!

When you are caring for others daily, take that gentle talk, that tough-love approach, that patient direction and use it on yourself. These techniques may not change how great you are at work, but they will no doubt open your eyes to the needs of caring for the number one person in your life with just as much love as you do for others.

As a licensed massage therapist for over 30 years, I fully understand the ramifications and sacrifices caregivers go through while taking care of other people. They are called to make someone else feel safe and pain-free even on their own worst days, when they themselves are struggling with bodily pain, emotional discomfort, and mental exhaustion. Even on days when they are at their worst, they still must buck up and go to work to heal others' bodies, minds, and souls.

Even before the worldwide COVID-19 pandemic struck us all, I was determined to write this book for all the nurses, doctors, first responders, parents, massage therapists, veterans and their families, teachers, and anybody else who has ever found themselves in the position of caretaker.

My hope is to inspire communities to commune, get stronger and reach out: that's the only real plan that can build resiliency in a society and in the people around us. If you are a caregiver or know one, share these strategies with others. It is always best to share any knowledge you have with others! When we act from a place of sharing and community rather than selfishness and competition, we truly embody the mindset of the caregiver. How many times have you heard the flight attendant explain, "In the event of a loss of cabin pressure, the oxygen mask will drop; be sure to put your mask on yourself first before assisting others!" That is what this book is about: self-care is *essential*. To be more effective, happier, more resilient, and less resentful in your own life, we must start "at home."

CHAPTER 1

SELF-CARE:
THE HOW'S AND WHY'S

"I was so busy building gardens I did not enjoy the one I was standing in!"
— Tamron Hall

The World Health Organization (WHO) Trusted Source defines self-care as: *"The ability of individuals, families and communities to promote health, prevent disease, maintain health, and to cope with illness and disability with or without the support of a healthcare provider."*

Who needs to focus on self-care? Well, over the years it has become abundantly clear that we *all* do. **However, in the wake of events like the COVID-19 pandemic, the world is beginning to understand the importance of essential workers and their need to stay healthy, happy, and whole.** Their well-being is critical to maintaining the well-being of all the rest of us!

During the lockdown, I became a "happy hermit." I realized that driving 33,000 miles a year, battling traffic, being late, flat tires, tolls, gas prices, and piling stress upon stress upon stress did *not* need to be my reality. At the same time, my clients realized that I could be just as effective remotely and I will never turn back. I learned who my real friends were, and I also learned that I needed to carve out time to cultivate a handful of beautiful friendships instead of wasting a bucketful of time on people who added nothing to my life.

You may not have the option of working from home — post-pandemic, many have had to return to their busy schedules — but that makes it all the more important for you to employ daily self-awareness and care. This book is here to lay it all out for you, to inspire you with ideas you never thought of, to encourage you to take yourself seriously and choose *you* first. I promise it will be worth it to create a life that is more enjoyable to live and filled with purpose. My mission for you is to encourage you to engage in easy, accessible, and meaningful practices to illuminate your life. This book is meant to be a "tool for life" to help you stop the cycle and start your journey to a fulfilling life.

SELF-CARE CHALLENGES FOR ESSENTIAL WORKERS

If you're an essential caregiver, it may seem to you that others can glide through life with grace and ease, defying pressures. The truth is that, in every town and every city in the world, there are countless people who are frustrated yet do not know where to turn. They fall into traps of pain, suffering, depression and ultimate dis-ease.

The differences in the lives of people deemed essential workers run very deep. It's not that they suffer more than others, or more frequently. **It's more subtle than that, hence why it all too often goes ignored or unnoticed.** Most people go to work and know what the daily to-do list entails. They know the goals, they have deadlines to get things done, and they get to enjoy that feeling you get when your lists are complete.

True essential workers do not have that same luxury. While they start the day similarly to everyone else, they have unique challenges that need to be understood and honored. As a nurse, for example, you'll go to work and while you may start out doing paperwork, in a flash the emergency room can fill up with unspeakable tragedy, the pace increases a hundredfold, and split decisions need to be made. Heart rates go up, and some days deep sadness is the end result.

This is a prime example of why self-care is essential.

According to Psychology Today,* self-care is related to better mental health:

Self-care is a commitment to ourselves, a promise to factor ourselves into the equation of our lives. When we optimize self-care, we feel better, look better, and have more energy. And quality self-care is linked to improved mental health, with benefits like enhanced self-esteem and self-worth, increased optimism, a positive outlook on life, and lower levels of anxiety and depression. The road to self-sacrifice is paved with good intentions. We sacrifice ourselves to meet deadlines, help others, and show others we love and care for them by going above and beyond to help them. We over-extend, over-promise, and exhaust ourselves so often and so much that we don't even realize how tired and stressed we are.

Many people see self-care as too generous or extravagant, even selfish. Nothing could be further from the truth; taking care of yourself is actually critical for mental, emotional and physical health and welfare. There are many reasons I want to share to convince you to flip the script in your life and start taking better care of yourself:

YOU ARE WORTHY

Self-care is important to maintaining a healthy relationship with yourself as it produces positive feelings and boosts your confidence and self-esteem. Also, self-care is necessary to remind yourself and others that you and your needs are important. Being worthy should not be considered a special privilege; as humans, we are all worthy of love, community, help and happiness. **What is needed is for essential workers to see their own worth in the same terms that they see their patient's.** It's a two-way street. I know nurses that care for people with everything they have (including some people who are not even very nice), and while the nurse still sees them as worthy of the best care and their precious time, they don't hold the same as true for themselves.

---

*www.psychologytoday.com/us/blog/a-deeper-wellness/202302/understanding-the-mental-health-and-self-care-connection

LIFE SHOULD BE BALANCED

Being a workaholic is not a benefit, nor should it be considered a badge of honor. **Too much work results in stress and exhaustion and can actually make you less productive, scattered and mentally depleted.** This will ultimately lead to a multitude of health problems, like anxiety, depression, insomnia, and many other diseases. Think of the word disease and break it down DIS-EASE. People do not think that disease is caused by anything other than genetics but that is proven over and over to be wrong. As a matter of fact, only 5-10% of breast cancer in women is genetic. **Self-care means as much as you commit to work, you must pledge to downtime**, and there are only so many hours in a day, we cannot change that, as we read in the previous story. Set boundaries for yourself and mindfully account for the hours in a day that will keep you at your mental peak. This could mean actually taking your lunch break, taking a quick walk after you eat before going back to work, stop working to spend quality time with people you love, and getting adequate rest and sleep at night, device-free.

STRESS MANAGEMENT MATTERS

Everybody has a little bit of stress. That's normal: our bodies are equipped to handle short bursts of stress.

Think of it like this: Imagine a caveman, just minding his own business. All of a sudden, he spots a saber-toothed tiger bearing down on him. What does he do? Well, first he drops what he's doing and makes a quick assessment of his safety, but more importantly, he runs as fast as he can! Once the threat was passed and the crisis averted, however, he returns to what he was doing without another thought.

Modern living has us in a constant slow drip stress situation all day, circumstances which weigh heavy on you and your health. Report deadlines are short-lived, an extra day of overbookings is rare, one skipped meal can be tolerated...but taken all together, the effect of these small, constant stressors is cumulative on the body. Go too long without relief, and you will start to break down.

If you sat for a minute right now I bet you could recall a time where the burden was too high and you had palpitations and you felt as though you could never catch your breath and the meal you just ate wreaked havoc on your stomach. Sound familiar?

I do not live in a world where I think we can wholly eliminate stress, but I do believe that consciously restructuring our lives, schedules, routines, and the people around us to lessen our burdens (while allotting special time for our own mental health) can help us to *properly* manage the stress that we cannot necessarily control. See Chapter 4 for goal-setting techniques to help you achieve better management of time and stress.

YOU SHOULD BE ENJOYING LIFE TO THE FULLEST

On my walk to surgery, I realized that while I may not be in control of every single thing that happens in my life, I *was* the only one who could make it a happier life worth living. Most of us work, making the person in command richer and making others happy... and what does it get us? Resentment, sickness, burnout. Stop living according to the mantra that says, "Once I get _____, I will be happy;" instead, make your new mantra, "Once I am happy, I will achieve _____!"

I have a tattoo on my arm that reminds me that every day of my life is a gift to be treated with respect. **Today is the day you decide to improve the quality of your life so you can better take care of yourself and others.** I am not suggesting quitting your job or making hasty life changes, but rather carving out more time for yourself, prioritizing the things that need to get done against the things that should be done for yourself and deleting things off your list that will not help in creating a better life. You'll be surprised to see that world does not stop just because your work to-do list was not done all in one day. Small wonder that many countries in the world today have seen how longer lunches and more vacation time have actually made their employees *more* productive, despite less work hours.

Be efficient and clear with your day. Once you start these practices, you will find yourself enjoying days that are more balanced and have extra "me time." It is much easier to get out of bed when you're excited for the day ahead! For example: I make a point of getting up earlier so I can really enjoy my extra-large cup of coffee before embarking on my day; I look forward to it and it makes me more motivated in the long run. As a caregiver of someone, you have likely told your patients, friends, family, or clients that life is an irreplaceable and treasured gift, all the while ignoring that wisdom yourself, behind the scenes!

STARTING SELF-CARE

Self-care is about your mental, emotional, and physical self. You must eat well, move more, take time to be still. This book provides many simple strategies to enhance your life easily, including how to eat healthier, get adequate sleep, care about your hygiene, exercise regularly, and more.

What is self-care? According to the Oxford Dictionary:

self-care
/ˌselfˈker/
noun

1. the practice of taking action to preserve or improve one's own health. "Autonomy in self-care and insulin administration"
2. the practice of taking an active role in protecting one's own well-being and happiness, in particular during periods of stress.

There will be times when we need to press pause and take care of ourselves. The trick is figuring out 1) how to tell when it's time to take a break and 2) how to effectively reset and recharge our batteries. And it starts by appreciating how we all have the power to *decide* to live our lives in a way that supports and enhances our physical and mental health.

For example, before I could even think of writing this book and sharing ideas with you, I knew I could not help anybody authentically without my own self-care. "Expressing oneself is an essential form of self-care" is an idea I took to heart in creating this book.

This entails doing anything for yourself that brings joy or helps improve your mental and physical health, including:

Going for a walk or jog

Meditating

Deep breathing

Taking a break when you need it

Researching aromatherapy

Workouts and doing yoga

Setting daily goals and sticking to them

Stopping the mind chatter

Getting rid of excess chemical products in your home

Taking a day off or half day

Choosing who you spend time with

Laughing

Making good food choices

Getting more sleep

Learning to say "no"

PHYSICAL SELF-CARE

Physical health is a priority for proper self-care. Taking care of your body with proper nutrition and exercise not only feels good, but it will also change your overall mood. Proper and regular exercise increases the levels of serotonin in your body, the feel-good hormone. It is important to physically move your body several times a day to take advantage of that distinct connection between body and mind, increasing energy and mood at the same time. When you consider an exercise routine in accordance with your commitment to self-care, you should always choose something that you actually like to do.

There are many options, and you should try several until you figure out what brings you joy and makes you motivated to actively participate in each day. **I start with the idea of "take five;"** instead of becoming overwhelmed with the information I am laying out and strategizing about how to fit it all in, I just take five. What this trains me to do is allocate just a few minutes here or there to incorporate something physical I enjoy, which in turn helps me better perform at my original task. It doesn't need to be five minutes on the dot; try walking, jogging, running, or yoga for 10, 15, 30 minutes. Turn on your favorite music and dance for half an hour, take a dip in a pool for 20 minutes, lift weights for a little while...to name just a few. **When you find the activity that you love, you are more likely to stick to a regimen and succeed at proper self-care.** You do not even have to join the gym to achieve a proper workout; these days, you can go online and find coaching for virtually anything for free or nominal fees.

SLEEP

Most people today are precariously sustaining their crazy, hectic lives on horribly insufficient amounts of sleep. This can be very detrimental to the quality of your life and ability to perform your best at your job. Essential workers do not have the luxury of going to work tired and laying back, after all. They must be on point all the time at a moment's notice! I know I would not want to think that my American Troops are too tired, demoralized or frustrated by their lives to perform their work. **Even people who think they are getting enough hours of sleep do not realize that their sleep is not of the quality needed to sustain health.** Studies suggest people get an average of 6–8 hours of sleep every night. (I have also always benefitted from an afternoon nap, but that is not always an option, so we must count on proper rest at night.) Later in this book, I will guide you through some options of meditation and aromatherapy to help aid your night routine.

DIET AND NUTRITION

Eating is as important as the preceding ideas to make you a better, happier employee and most productive and healthy. **Junk goes into the body; junk comes out of the body—it's as simple as that**. When you are running ragged, you often forget to eat and then, when blood sugar levels are so out of whack, you grab the first thing you can get a hold of and binge on junk or excess coffee to get by. Eating healthy and balanced with the recommended guidelines of fats, protein, and carbohydrates, you will quickly see the difference in your productivity, sleep, and mood. I will suggest several on-the-go snacks and eating options to help optimize your busy life.

SOCIAL SELF-CARE

What I have become acutely aware of during the isolation in the 2020 pandemic was that much of my overscheduled time was spent with people that I did not want to be around, and long hours in my car wasted time and added undue stress. **I was not being efficient enough with my time to be able to address my own needs.** I realized how I wanted to set goals for being home more, because this made me happy, then back-tracked how I could achieve this goal and took action each day.

TIME MANAGEMENT

I now drive less (from 33,000 miles a year to less than 2,000), have a shorter workweek, and allow more time for personal care. This has become sacred to me; even if I could book more appointments, I know my earning goals for the week that make me comfortable and I reach them, no more and no less. I created personal boundaries and I stick to it. This may seem easy, but it is challenging to stay the course putting me on the front burner.

What part of your day do you dread? How can you change that to live happier? **You must live on purpose, being methodical about who, what, and where you are each day.** I will help you understand how to set goals in your life, achieve them, and stick to them.

Along with goals, you need to understand that, even if you are doing a job that does not give you complete pleasure, you are not alone, and that makes it even more important to carve out time each day for the things that bring you pleasure.

SAYING "THANK YOU" AND SAYING "NO"

Daily practice of gratitude is another important way to help boost your mood and make you feel better. Research by UC Davis psychologist Robert Emmons, author of *Thanks! How the New Science of Gratitude Can Make You Happier*, shows that simply keeping a gratitude journal — regularly writing brief reflections on moments for which we're thankful — can significantly increase well-being and life satisfaction.

Your gratitude practice does not have to be a big deal, just regularly practiced. I write each day in my calendar 1–3 things that I am grateful for, from my health to fresh cookies. It is easy and astounding how peaceful you will be when you realize, no matter what your circumstances are, you have much to be grateful for. **Prioritizing gratitude time as well as meditation or regular mindfulness practice are imperative to**

mood, better living, and enhanced health. I will take you through user-friendly techniques to employ each day, whether you are on the move or lying down and in deep relaxation. When you start to use these techniques on a daily basis you are living a life overflowing with self-care.

In order to make time for *you* and self-care, you must learn to say "no" more. This is a concept that was very difficult for me; I was told to never say no, to take every opportunity because you never know where it will go. I did that for a while and was spread thin, resentful, and overwrought with lengthy to-do lists each day. Even when I completed a 30-point list in a day, I never felt as though I accomplished anything. I now trust my gut and never give an answer right away. I take time to consider the pros and cons of every opportunity that comes my way. **Even if it is a great opportunity, it may not be the best use of my time in alignment with where I want my life to go and my goals.** So, consider that. Do not say yes in order to pacify others' feelings; we are beyond that now! That way of living is detrimental to your self-care. Be grateful for the offer, consider it fully and make informed decisions.

What I should be crystal clear about is how you choose to live your life and what you do for self-care is utterly up to you, without judgment from others, or guilt conjured up in your head, or by the values instilled in you when you grew up. This is your life to be lived your way, enough said. Just the way you have never let your patients, clients, country, and family down, now it's the time to not let *you* down!

IMPROVING SELF-AWARENESS

All of the techniques in this book are for the sole purpose of increasing your awareness of the quality of your life and to increase your strength to handle life in a more welcoming way. We want to eliminate the constant fight-or-flight response of heavy breathing, frenetic movement and higher blood pressure and replace it with more time in the relaxation mode. **Relaxation mode is lower blood pressure and heart rate, increased digestive rate, clearer thinking, and less stress hormones.**

A person in tune with their body may feel their mood changes, sleep suffers, and their productivity goes down when they are in these types of work environments. A study conducted in Great Britain and published in the Journal of Affective Disorders analyzed data from half a million women and men, aged 37–73 years old. The study subjects reported that they spend two and half hours outdoors daily, while researchers found that each additional hour spent outside in natural light was linked to a corresponding decrease in the risk of developing long-term depression.

Do not be intimidated by the thought of adding two and half hours outside, just take five, start there. Consider taking a moment outside, carve out time, cut down on the blue light in your bedroom, and do not bring your phone into the bedroom. In a 2018 study, people who slept with very low levels of background light in their bedroom had double the risk of depression over a five-year period compared to those who slept in pitch darkness. This seems like an easy way to start to improve our mental health.

We need to start by taking action. Reading this book and considering that you currently do not care enough for yourself is a good step, but no goal ever is attained by just thinking — you must act. **Just because you own a candle does not mean it will light up your life; there are steps you take to ensure it does its job. The same goes for your own life.** Get the match, strike it, carefully light the wick and there you have it. Before you initiate any of the techniques, I suggest you take my five senses approach to your own home or workspace.

ENGAGING THE SENSES

We all know the five senses: sight, smell, taste, touch, and hearing. What's needed now is to learn how to engage them in your personal spaces to better enjoy yourself and settle in.

SIGHT

Let's start with sight. Make sure each and every thing on your desk and in every room is something useful to you and/or makes you totally happy and inspired. For example, I have a magnetic board over my desk which I rearrange at least quarterly with great pictures that I love, cool goals, cut out magazine pictures, and amazing quotes. This way, if I ever sit back in frustration, arms folded, I can look up and see all these great things that make me delighted. I often go room by room and rearrange, get rid of, and question each thing to make my space peaceful. If there is an object in your room that you do not like, perhaps because someone gave it to you instead of you having chosen it, consider getting rid of it. You may have obligations at work, but your sacred space exists only to make you happy, not to dredge up old negative feelings of people or situations.

Another aspect of sight in relation to your health is literally how you light your home. **Research shows that an adequate amount of light improves mood and energy levels, while poor lighting contributes to depression and other deficiencies in the body.** The amount and type of lighting directly affects concentration, appetite, mood, and many other aspects of daily life. Scientists think that nighttime exposure to blue light throws off your sleep/wake cycle, leading to symptoms of depression. That's because your circadian rhythm plays a role in several brain and behavioral processes, like neurotransmission and hormone secretion. Along similar lines, most people see little to no natural light in their personal workspace — especially in places like police precincts, schools, and hospitals. While you cannot change that, you *can* make time to take three deep breaths outside in natural light.

Another option is to research how different color bulbs relate to emotions. My desk has a low green light to help with my migraines, but the light is so soothing and soft at the same time — it just makes me feel good!

SMELL

Now let's consider the sense of smell. Just as you went around the home and workplace and definitively decided to keep only the things you love or use, your surroundings must smell good. When a scent makes it to your brain through the nose, it releases feel-good endorphins and serotonin. These can improve your mood, giving you mental clarity and easing your tension.

Think about a time you were driving along and drove by a recently hit skunk (we have all been there). What happens to your body? You immediately tense up; your face squishes, you hold your breath, increasing your anxiety and heart rate. This is an extreme example, but any bad smell, small or large, does this to your body. This can even happen to the point that you get so used to smells that you do not smell them anymore — how good can that be? Smell is important, so bring a plant to clear the surrounding air, keep a subtle candle burning, or have a cotton ball soaked in essential oil tucked in your desk. I will also teach you more about aromatherapy in Chapter 6.

TASTE

Taste is a little less obvious. Scientists are saying that the way we react to things that we find objectionable is all based originally on foods that we don't like the taste of. We often use the phrase "it left a bad taste in my mouth" to describe an activity or a situation that we find quite unpleasant. But now, researchers writing in the Journal of Science have shown that there may be more to this metaphor than meets the eye.

The researchers, led by Hannah Chapman, wondered if there was any kind of link between the facial movements made when we eat disgusting food and when we see disgusting pictures or when we experience unpleasant behavior. To start with, the researchers gave volunteers different drinks that were either neutral tasting, sweet or bitter. They then took close video images of their faces, focusing on the actions of a group of muscles called the levator labii as well as other facial muscles that make us wrinkle up our noses and raise our upper lips when we taste something nasty. Unsurprisingly, they found that the bitter taste caused a big movement of these muscles compared to sweet or neutral tastes.

Next, the scientists showed people pictures of disgusting things (including feces, injuries, insects, things like that) and compared these with pictures of sad things, alongside some neutral pictures for contrast. The team found that only the disgusting pictures led to the movement of these facial muscles, and the stronger the disgust that the person felt, the more their muscles moved. This was quite intriguing, and the team went on to look at situations where people experienced unpleasant or unfair situations. These were met with these same facial movements of disgust seen with a nasty liquid or unpleasant pictures.

The researchers concluded that moral disgust and outrage actually have similar evolutionary roots to physical disgust, and they think that this physical response to something nasty has probably been co-opted during our social evolution to express our disgust at social and moral situations that we don't like.

FAKING A SMILE

Consider the study published by Linda Johnson on visiblebody.com in "The science behind a (fake) smile."

Even if you're not actually happy, activating the muscles associated with smiling can fool your brain into thinking you are. Lead researcher Sarah Pressman PhD of the University of Kansas explains, "It's not just that our brains are happy and make us smile, it can also be the opposite—we feel the smile and become happy."

The muscles of expression located around the mouth are the depressor anguli oris, therisorius, the zygomaticus major, the zygomaticus minor, and the levator labii superioris. All of these muscles, specifically the zygomaticus muscles, are involved with smiling; they pull the orbicularis oris (the circular muscle of your mouth) upwards. These muscles are innervated by the various branches of the facial nerve (VII), which—when the muscles are activated—send signals to the brain that you are smiling.

From there, endorphins are released into the bloodstream from the pituitary gland and the brain and spinal cord from the hypothalamus. Endorphins are opioids (chemicals that bind to opiate receptors) peptides that act as neurotransmitters. Think of endorphins as the body's natural painkillers, or opiates; they are released in times of stress (good and bad), exercise, excitement, pain, love, and other emotional states, and you feel awesome because of them. If you've ever smiled helplessly at a picture of a puppy or kitten, you're feeling the effects of endorphins.

But how do these endorphins affect not only your state of mind, but also your heart rate? **Simple: if your brain believes it is feeling happiness, you will not be stressed, or at least will be less stressed than you would be if you were unhappy.**

> Now imagine these stress-easing tactics used over a long-term period. This is what was measured in the University of Michigan study. 9% may not seem like that much of a drop in risk levels, but when you stack it against all the other variables one can encounter in life, it's a significant decrease. So, the next time you're in the middle of a heated argument, or bad taste, smile for self-care.

TOUCH

What about touch? Most people who have experienced an amazing massage, a great hug, or a comfy blanket, can remember how all those things made them feel. Now think of the itchy sweater, a hard chair, or an ill-fitting shoe. These are all experiences with touch. Making sure all your clothes feel good on your body, shoes are the right size, and the fabrics on your furnishings and bedding are the best they can be for you, all contribute to a general sense of well-being, comfort and reassuring control over your immediate environment. Essential workers are often called to wear specific uniforms that can induce negative feelings, and while you cannot change your uniform, you *can* make sure to change into comfortable, happiness-invoking garments the moment you get home! You can even consider upping your undergarment game to make you feel comfortable and attractive. **Receiving physical touch increases levels of dopamine and serotonin, two neurotransmitters that help normalize your mood and ease stress and anxiety.** Dopamine is also known to regulate the pleasure center in your brain that can offset feelings of anxiety, so make sure the things in your surroundings give you the best chance for relaxation. More on self-massage techniques to calm the cardiovascular system and trigger the release of oxytocin in Chapter 2.

HEARING

Lastly, your sense of hearing. In *The Hidden Messages in Water*, author Masaru Emoto discovered how sounds affect water's structure. Water can absorb and store sound effects, and, using an electron microscope, Emoto showed how much frozen water's structure depends on the sounds absorbed. For example, after one hour of praying, the structure of water — rather than appearing as a shapeless blob, looked like a smooth, beautiful, and perfect six-rayed snowflake. This transformation takes place because of the precise pronunciation of the speaker's voice, creating sound pressure that is equal to the frequency of the magnetic field of the Earth (8 dB).

As humans are approximately 60 percent water, the import of Emoto's experiments can be crucial to our physical well-being.

For your well-being, carefully consider what you listen to on the radio; what you watch on TV while drinking your coffee; who you choose to have conversations with; and the words that come out of your own mouth. I would like to suggest playing certain sounds and frequencies in your home while you go about your day. More specifically, solfeggio frequencies.

Solfeggio frequencies are a set of healing tones dating back to the 11th century which have been used in a variety of cultures for their potential healing properties. Just as many cultures today believe certain sound waves can heal, it is believed that the specific syllables associated with notes can have an impact on the body and our emotions. These specific sound waves can penetrate deep into the subconscious mind and activate the repairing processes of the body on a cellular level to treat ailments such as pain, depression, and anxiety. This is in alignment with many of the emotions felt by essential workers that need to be addressed. Solfeggio frequencies also have a variety of physical and mental health benefits, ranging from helping to coordinate brain waves to promoting and helping to repair relationships.

Listening to Solfeggio frequencies for even ten minutes twice a week can enable the body to manifest a range of healing benefits, including:

- Pain and stress relief (174Hz)
- Tissue and organ healing (285Hz)
- Free yourself from guilt and fear (396Hz)
- Facilitate change (417Hz)
- Activate intuition and affect well-being (528Hz)
- Facilitate relationships (639Hz)
- Problem solving by the gut (741Hz)
- Balance your spirituality (852Hz)
- Enlightenment (963Hz)

CONCLUDING THOUGHTS

I hope now you have a deeper understanding of the importance of tending to your life and surroundings via the five senses. It always blows my mind how often people go through their day so numb to feelings of the senses. The preceding ideas are simple yet can make a huge impact on the way you experience life going forward. Now that we have a solid foundation about how to stimulate the five senses, change perspective on our surroundings and feelings on a less direct level, I am moving on to how to create physical change in your body through manual manipulation and massage. In order to fully explore benefits of self-care, it is important to understand every way we can achieve it.

CHAPTER 2

SELF-MASSAGE TECHNIQUES

In the previous chapter, we discussed the importance of engaging the senses to practice proper self-care. Of the five senses, touch is arguably the most important — it literally affects the way we "feel" at any given time. And one of the greatest (I'm not biased, I swear!) ways of leveraging the sense of touch to relax and rejuvenate is with a massage.

Massages can relax your muscles, relieve stress, boost your energy... the list goes on. **But would you believe you don't need a professional massage therapist to ease your pain?**

And a good thing, too; your busy schedule as a caregiver does not usually allow you the extra time to book a massage with a licensed massage therapist. Even if you did, you'd probably end up needing to cancel it anyway after some unforeseen emergency.

That's why this chapter is all about avoiding suffering in your day-to-day life through the use of self-massage techniques that can fit into anyone's schedule. They are virtually free and are best done in the privacy of your own home. This type of self-care consumes less time, giving you *more* time to spend on your specific problem areas, rather than the broader spectrum routines of massaging the body many therapists thoughtlessly go through. For essential caregivers, we'll be focusing on self-massage techniques that can be implemented with your fingers, hands, and elbows, or using tools such as tennis balls, foam rollers, and golf balls.

CHALLENGES FOR CAREGIVERS

Caregivers often experience extremely long workdays where they are not allowed to be in tune with their bodies until the workday is over. Then, as soon as they punch out, they come face to face with pain, discomfort, and issues that can only inhibit the quality of their work. In order to target these chronic areas of discomfort, you need to work your **trigger points—knots and bulges in the muscle tissues that can cause pain and refer pain to other areas of the body due to pressurizing the nerves.**

In my experience being a massage therapist since 1990, my clients that incorporate self-massage between appointments (combined with exercise) saw a reduction in their pain intensity and had more enjoyable, pain-free daily activities.

BESIDES FEELING GREAT, SELF-MASSAGE CAN HAVE SEVERAL BENEFITS, INCLUDING:

- Pain reduction
- Less missed work
- Better focus on the job
- Reduced swelling, edema, and soreness
- Reduced anxiety and stress
- Revitalized bodies
- Improved sleep

Like massage in general, self-massage may help several reasons for pain and discomfort, including stress, anxiety, headaches, digestive/stomach issues, muscle tension, foot pain, hand pain, and more. When combined as part of a comprehensive treatment plan, self-massage can also help manage other conditions like fibromyalgia, poor circulation, or arthritis. It should not replace regular medical care. **Self-massage may extend the benefits and provide relief in between trained professional sessions.** Self-massage may ease many types of minor pain, like head, neck, shoulders, belly, back, and hand pain. The techniques that I will share

are simple to do anywhere. It is best to use cream to reduce skin friction. You can even add these massage tips to your daily shower routine.

The idea is to be proactive to pain, not reactive when it is acute. Try a quick full-body massage technique to stimulate circulation and wake you up when you start to feel sluggish and reach for your fourth cup of coffee. Referred to as a "tapotement" type of action, it's a great choice to release muscle tension quickly and easily. Make a gentle fist and use the pinky side of the fist. This type of body work may be particularly helpful for firefighters, service people, and police officers, jobs that — due to their nature of protecting the public and providing service to others — come with a lot of opportunities to increase overall tension in the body.

Start with your lower legs and arms nearest your hands, and gently apply a light blow to your lower legs, calves, hamstrings, and thighs. Move to your torso and do the same from the lower abdomen up, complete to the arms and wherever you can reach. Always move toward the midline of the body and toward the heart rather than the fingers. This goes for any massage. Do not hit too hard and cause bruising; apply enough pressure behind the blows that make a difference in regard to your tension, not so much you create another problem, especially if you bruise easily. The tapping-like action delivers a light blow to stimulate the area and increase circulation; you should aim to have the fist bounce off the body part. You can repeat as many times as you need until you can feel the vibration and buzzing of a revitalized body.

AS INCREDIBLE AS ALL THIS MAY SOUND, YOU SHOULD KEEP A FEW THINGS IN MIND:

1. You need not set aside an hour; you may only need a few minutes to get satisfying results.

2. You can revisit chronic pain areas several times a day.

3. You may need to feel around a bit to find the root of the pain; it is not always where you think.

4. Play around with the pressure you use if you want to feel relief, not create more soreness.

5. Consider using in conjunction with several of the yoga stretches in this book for the best results.

NECK

One of the most frequent problem areas of the body part is the neck. The neck is often slumped forward due to hours of focus at a computer or on a phone and this can create tension and tightness. Neck tension is also a by-product seen in nurses who have to lift and move patients; doctors who are zoned in on a patient in surgery; and dental professionals who often find themselves in slumped positions. Another reason your neck can give you issues is that, when we are stressed and busy, the tendency is to squeeze the shoulders up toward your ears, again creating tightness in the top of the shoulders and trapezius muscles that can cause pain, tension headaches, impaired comfort when sleeping, and gradually decrease the mobility of the neck. Make a point of giving your neck frequent breaks during the day to provide relief from hunching over your computer, staring at your phone or tablet, and the poor postural habits referred to nowadays as **tech neck.**

TARGETED SELF-MASSAGE FOR NECKS

Start by doing 1–3 minutes of inhale/exhale shoulder shrugs to release tension and bring some heat to the neck and shoulders. I start most yoga classes with this move for 1–3 minutes, and people immediately feel looser and more heated!

Follow this by turning the head to the right and left while keeping your chin parallel to the floor, then add right-to-left rotations with the chin slightly lowered. Continue this movement for 1–3 minutes. Next, try lateral movements; sit up tall, shoulders down, and drop your right ear to your right shoulder, inhale through center, and left ear toward the left shoulder. Finally, for the neck warm-up, maintaining the tall straight back drop your chin to chest center and lift the chin to the sky. Take caution when lifting your chin so as not to feel pinching in the back of the neck.

Now we can start some self-massage!

Clasp your hands together behind your neck with your pinkies up against the base of your skull and apply pressure to each side of your neck with the bottom of your palms. Rub up and down slowly, and squeeze and release the pressure of the hands to the side of the neck. It is important not to squeeze too hard or for too long along the carotid artery to maintain proper blood flow to the brain.

Place the fingertips of your right hand in a firm position and press into the left side of the cervical spine (the muscles laying adjacent to the vertebra). Press the tips of your fingers into all the tight areas, then take the right fingers and apply firm pressure into the trapezius muscle, or top edge of the shoulders, along the left side of your neck just under the base of your skull, walking the fingers out to the top of the shoulder. If you feel a spot that seems to be offering great relief, hang there for a bit and gently persuade the musculature or do a little digging. Be careful if you have long nails; if that is the case, use the pads of your fingers (where you would find your fingerprint).

While burrowing the fingers around and into your tension, rock your head from left to right. Repeat this as many times as you need on each side, noting that each side is different, and one side may need more attention than the other.

As a side note, many people forget the front of the neck which can hold just as much tension when your head is held static for hours at your desk, on the phone, or even driving. It's best to use more caution when stretching the front neck and massaging because of the arteries, as it can cause pinching when tipping the chin up. So pay attention! You can also slide down in your desk chair and rest the base of the skull on the top of the chair back. The pressure will continue to open the back of your neck while the stretch in the anterior neck will stimulate your thyroid glands and relieve tension. Rock the head left to right and hold on to any juicy spots.

SHOULDERS AND ARMS

Poor posture and hunching at a desk all day can also lead to rounded shoulders and deep, debilitating shoulder pain. **The continuous tension which essential workers endure on normal workdays easily ends up being carried in their shoulders, subsequently radiating down into the arms.** Careers like nursing home care, firefighting, service men and women, and surgical nurses, which involve carrying heavy equipment but which are also subject to extreme focus, can lead to worsening shoulder stiffness and pain going ignored or unnoticed until it becomes acute. Unaddressed shoulder pain and stiffness can lead to a loss of range of motion and clogging in the armpit nodes.

TARGETED SELF-MASSAGE FOR SHOULDERS AND ARMS

Take the fingers of your right hand over your left shoulder; your palm will cup the top of your shoulders. Gently start to squeeze, pinch firmly, and move your fingers in circular motions on any dense bumps you may feel; you will know when you hit it. Remember the other side.

Work, stress, and hours of driving can create a lot of tension in the arms. **This type of tension, unaddressed over time, will travel up to the shoulders and beyond, so stay on it even if you do not feel pain, remember to be proactive.** Moving and manipulating the muscles in your arms will release tension, increase circulation, and speed up recovery.

Start with your right hand on your left wrist and systematically pinch, squeeze and knead the muscles of the forearms past the elbow to the upper arm and shoulder, pay attention to the fleshy areas rather than the bones. Do this several times at all arm angles; remember to work from your fingertips toward the heart for best results, and to encourage lymph drainage in the hands for better circulation. In the end, take your left arm above the elbow and pull it across your chest; take a deep breath and feel the great stretch. Repeat on the other side.

Once you complete each side, wrap your arms around your chest as though you were hugging yourself, and if possible, lock your fingertips around the inner edge of the shoulder blades, take several deep breaths and gently lift the elbows and lower the elbows several times. You can even hold the shoulder blades and bend the torso left to right or all directions. Uncross the arms and repeat this move with the other arm stacked on top; the side that is not your habit will feel weird.

HANDS

Sitting and typing all day, writing, tight grips, lifting equipment and driving can all wreak havoc on the hands, creating pain and tension. This type of tension can lead to weakness and carpal tunnel problems. **Any essential worker can benefit from better hand circulation for grip and mobility, especially the many categories of caregivers who find themselves contributing hours at a desk to update logs and case files.**

TARGETED SELF-MASSAGE FOR HANDS

Start by opening and closing your hands into tight fists and spreading your fingers. Spread the fingers apart so wide you feel the stretch into the palm. This movement helps warm up the fascia and release excess lymph from the fingers. If your hands feel particularly stiff doing this, consider holding your hands above the heart for 1–3 minutes to move the lymph along. Interlace your fingers, apply pressure, and do circles with the wrist joints and bottom of the palms.

Next, take your right thumb and start firm circles of pressure at the base of the left thumb and along the base of and between each finger, do not be afraid to press it will feel great. Squeeze each finger from the tip of the finger to the base a few times each. Rub the webbing between each finger, and to finish, stretch each finger apart from its neighbor, then repeat on the other hand. A great time to get in the habit of this self-care practice is when you are applying hand cream. This type of break in your day is more rejuvenating than you think!

STOMACH

Never thought of massaging your stomach? **In fact, a gentle abdomen massage can help stimulate digestion and deter constipation.** The abdomen is also affected when posture is poor. For essential care workers, it's not unusual to hold stress in their stomach resulting in inadequate digestion. Not to mention, their busy (and often unpredictable) schedules can lead to poor nutrition and inconsistent eating habits. We will talk more about that later in the chapter on nutrition.

TARGETED SELF-MASSAGE FOR STOMACHS

Using one or both palms, and the first three fingers, rub your abdomen in a clockwise circle. You should always start with your right lower abdomen, move up to approximately the belly button level, go across to the left, and then down. This movement is the way your digestion moves. This massage can relieve cramps, bloat, discomfort, and lower belly stiffness.

When using your hand or palm, continue gentle pressure and continuous circles, and when you get in a little deeper with your pointer, middle finger, and ring finger, you can press in and execute small deep circles with the fingers. This can be done sitting; however, for better results, lie down so you can apply deeper pressure. Try having the knees bent and feet flat to give you more slack in the belly area. These types of massages provide relief by stimulating a bowel movement. It can also reduce bloating, cramps, and abdominal tightness.

FEET

One of the most satisfying areas to massage are your feet. In addition to the feel-good aspect, **massaging the feet stimulates acupressure points corresponding to the whole body**, so if you must choose where to self-massage due to time, it is probably best to go for the soles. It goes without saying that nurses, doctors — in fact, caretakers of all types — are constantly on their feet, standing up and straining their legs and hips for hours on end.

TARGETED SELF-MASSAGE FOR FEET

For tense feet, place the bottom of your foot on a golf ball or lacrosse ball and use a wall to help you balance. (You always have the option of sitting to do this, but the pressure will be less.) Increasingly put more and more weight on the foot as the ball presses into your sole. Carefully move your foot in all directions until you feel a tender or stiff spot, then hold.

Please pay attention to the ball of the feet and heel, as they tend to take the most abuse during your day.

Once you have spent enough time on the bottoms of the feet, it is time to move to the toes. Just like when you worked your hands, start squeezing and rolling your toes individually with your fingers from tip to base.

Next, spread each toe apart from its neighbor and bend each toe forward and back. A technique I have used for decades when teaching my yoga classes and professional athletes is toe threading. This can significantly help sideline foot cramping, fascial stiffness, and tendonitis issues on the bottom of the foot.

While sitting comfortably and using your right hand, take hold of your left foot. Interlace one finger between each toe and try to get the base of the fingers all the way to the base of the toes in time. Your palm should be up against the bottom of the foot and hold this for 2 minutes. While doing it, you may not feel much; however, once you release the fingers, you will instantly feel the difference. Do the same thing on the other side. Make a habit while watching TV to sideline foot pain before it ever becomes an issue.

CALVES

Walking all day can shorten your calf muscles and start to affect your gait and knees. **For caregivers tasked with carrying equipment, climbing stairs, or just staying on their feet all day, taking proper care of their calves can make a night-and-day difference in terms of soreness and stiffness.**

TARGETED SELF-MASSAGE FOR CALVES

Taking your right hand, start at the ankle of your left foot. Pinch and squeeze the whole calf, moving towards the knee; repeat this several times. Do this action again, but instead of grabbing the whole calf, hold, pinch, and squeeze the inside part of the calf, then the outside part of the calf. Finish with a few ankle rolls in each direction. Repeat on the other side.

IT BAND AND LEG

Most people, at some time or another, have felt stiffness associated with the iliotibial band (IT band). This is a large muscle that starts on your hip bone and runs outside your thigh to just past the knee joint.

TARGETED SELF-MASSAGE FOR THE IT BAND

This muscle tends to be sensitive, so many people cannot tolerate using a foam roller. If this is the case, start at your knee squeeze and knead your outer thigh working your way up to your hip bone. If you feel the skin pinch, try some cream to help with the excess friction. You can also use the heel of your hand to perform pressurized circles on the length of the IT band. Spend a little extra time on the outer knee. Do not rub on the outer hip bone, which can irritate the bursa sacs. This very easy technique can alleviate knee, hip, and leg stiffness and soreness.

BUTTOCKS AND HIP

Just as the IT band can tighten, so can the hip and glutes. **Sitting, intense exercise, and being on your feet all day can lead to disorder in the area.** The glutes and hips can be tender to dig into, so go in gently and progressively increase pressure as needed. When paying attention to the glutes, you must be careful not to sink too deep into the center and aggravate the sciatic nerve.

TARGETED SELF-MASSAGE FOR THE BUTTOCKS AND HIP

For this area, you can use a foam roller, a tennis ball, or any ball with a little give to it. If it is too intense, start these moves on a mattress or on an easy chair. Start seated, take the ball or roller under your butt cheek, and have your knees bent and feet flat. Displace some of the weight of your torso on your hands behind you, slightly leaning back. Try rolling the ball around the glute and down toward the upper back thigh. Roll in all directions, sink more and more as the tissue gives way. Stay mindful here so you do not go near the bursa or nerves. Remember the other side.

BACK

The most sought-after area for pain relief in the body is the back. The National Institute of Health estimates over 90 billion dollars are spent annually in the US on back pain relief techniques. That total rises to 134 billion if you include the neck, so some daily self-care before you need it would be time well-spent. In my experience, at one time or another almost all my clients have suffered from back pain. If you are working in a hospital on a hard floor all day, that can increase back strain and stiffness. Lifting heavy equipment can also increase back pain to acute levels, demanding you take action.

TARGETED SELF-MASSAGE FOR THE BACK

For back pain, you can simulate the work of a "ma roller" (therapeutic self-massage tool that I love and recommend) by putting two tennis/golf balls into the toe of a sock. Lie down on them so that the balls are pressing on the muscles on either side of the spine, with the bones of the spine between the covered balls. Relax into the balls and take as many breaths as you need to feel the muscles release and sink in, and the pain subside; this can take anywhere between 1–10 minutes per spot depending on how tense your muscles are.

Breathe deeply. Start at your lower spine and systematically move up toward the base of your skull. At first, if you are tight and tense, this can be very challenging, but with time and consistency, it will be quicker and hurt less. A no-equipment-necessary procedure to try involves starting in a seated position, taking your thumbs on the arc of the hip bones, and rubbing them in circles using decent pressure.

Next, move more toward the midline to the sacrum, the base of the spine and the keystone of your spinal column; therefore, it bears the brunt of pressure all day. Continue the thumb circles on the sacrum as deep as you can. If you feel extra tightness in any area, linger there until you feel a release. If you pay close enough attention, a muscle/tissue release will feel like your thumbs pressing into frozen butter until the butter is overtaken by the heat in your hands and gives way. Finally, if you have good balance and lying against a ball is too intense, you can put a tennis ball on the wall, lean into it and raise and lower your body against the tense muscles.

HEADACHE

As a chronic migraine sufferer, I know how quickly head pain and tension can ruin your sleep and day and even cause loss of work. **The idea is to try to pay attention to your face, head, and scalp always.** It is safe to say doctors and nurses who are reading charts and focusing on wounds and injuries can hold tension in the head; even essential workers who internalize emotions can suffer here.

TARGETED SELF-MASSAGE FOR HEADACHES

First, take your fingertips beside your nostrils and do five or six circles with pressure right on the cheekbones. Little by little, work your way to your ear and repeat a few times. Next, move above the cheekbone and do the same thing and then below the cheekbone. Always work from the nose outward. Continue this same movement right below the brow, on the brow, and above the brow, even doing it on the whole forehead. When working on and around the brow, be aware that many sinuses are here, so the area can be extra sensitive. Try this same movement at the base of the skull, which is where most tension starts. As a bonus, use your fingers to apply pressure and make circular motions on the bone behind the ear.

Next, take the palms of your hands on either side of the forehead and squeeze your head together. There is a type of joint called **sutures** in the skull, and when you apply pressure here, it can reduce pain. Do this suture squeeze on all areas of the skull: top, side, and bottom. It is extra nice if someone does it for you. You can add the neck and eyes massage techniques here to round out an excellent self-care practice.

Finally, a method I have used on my massage clients for decades involves taking your fingers, grabbing your earlobes and pulling down. Move up the outer edges of the ears, squeeze and pull away from the skull. Do this for 20–30 rounds on each ear. Not only does this relieve tension, but it also brings a surge of blood and oxygen to the ears (you will know, as they will get red and hot). This is an amazing practice if you feel a cold coming on to beat it before it gets you. Then, interlace your fingers with the palms of your hands behind your head and drop your chin to chest center. Hold this stretch for three deep breaths, drop the right ear to your right shoulder and use your right hand on the upper left side of your skull. Stretch there for three breaths, repeat to the left, and finish with a few neck circles in each direction.

EYES

Tension headaches and eye strain are very prevalent in essential workers. The high stress levels, hours of writing charts or reports, and incredible time demands contribute to pressure in the eyes or head.

TARGETED SELF-MASSAGE FOR EYES

Here's a practice I encourage at the end of my yoga classes that helps bring healing heat to the eyes through the optic nerve to the brain, enables relaxation and eye strain after staring at screens all day. Vigorously rub your hands together until the palms heat up, then cup one hand over each eye to let the warmth soothe them. The circle of the palm gently pressing into the orbital bone of the eye socket also stimulates many acupressure points for relief and relaxation.

I like to do this at my desk and rest my head in my hands with my elbows on my desk, taking three long deep breaths. Finally, with your eyes gently closed, starting with your eyes in the 12 o'clock position, perform large circles to the right 10–15 times, then repeat to the left. Try all different movement patterns; I encourage my students to go left to right, up and down, the letter Z, and backward letter Z. This type of eye movement is easy and quick and can strengthen the eye muscles and improve vision.

EARTHING

If you do not have the time or desire to start a self-massage routine, a great way to reset the body is by **earthing**. Every care-giver who cannot find the time to employ these techniques and needs a quick fix in the energetic alignment in their body should give this a try. Not only will you get fresh air, but you will also be healing your body.

Earthing, also known as **grounding**, is the practice of connecting your body to the natural electrical charge of the earth. Earthing is as easy and available as walking barefoot outside, lying on a beach, and swimming in the ocean or a lake (not a pool). The earth is rich in free electrons (which carry a negative charge) that, when united to the body, can neutralize free radicals, delivering antioxidant and immune-boosting properties. A 2020 review study found that grounding had significant anti-inflammatory effects.*

Benefits of grounding include:

- Reduced fatigue
- Increased energy
- Reduced chronic pain
- Reduced inflammation
- Faster recovery from exercise
- Enhanced/elevated mood and improved depression
- Improved skin quality
- Reduced blood pressure and hypertension
- Support heart health
- Improved sleep quality

* www.sciencedirect.com/science/article/pii/S1550830719305476

As mentioned before, grounding is easy and free. Most people ground outdoors, taking their shoes and socks off, as it is best with direct skin contact and standing on bare earth, rock, or grass. Placing your hands on the earth and lying down are also effective. Consider taking this time for yourself after work, during lunch, or in the morning for 15–30 minutes daily. The healing qualities of this practice are ancient and astounding. Regular practice can even improve sleep for overworked caregivers.

Self-massage is suitable if you have mild to moderate pain. **But if the pain is intense or ongoing, feels like electric shocks, or extra deep, it is best to see a qualified therapist or doctor first.** Do not self-massage a break in a bone, wounds, or burns, do not go deep if you have thin skin. Never linger on bulging veins. Use your intuition, and stay tuned in.

Get medical attention if the pain worsens, doesn't get better, or you develop new symptoms. Your doctor can determine what's causing your pain and the best treatment for your situation. The best thing about these techniques is they can be done over your clothes and at work to relieve pain and stiffness before it gets bad and not to mention give you an energy boost.

CHAPTER 3
NUTRITIONAL SELF-CARE

A fundamental way to care for yourself is by nurturing your body with proper nutrients. I am not a nutritionist, and I am not going to reinvent the wheel; however, I *have* tried virtually every method of eating that there is for the benefit of my clients, so I'm at least speaking from experience! I want to offer you user-friendly options to choose from, while keeping it simple. What I know for sure is, no matter what anybody has done or told you, your body is individual with its own needs and set of circumstances. Stay the course, be honest with yourself, and most of all be kind to yourself with whatever mode of eating you choose.

As with any advice you may read, consult your doctor before drastically changing your eating habits. **Keep in mind when you maintain a diet of nutrient-rich foods, you are supporting your body, which will lead to experiencing fewer mood swings, better focus, and increased energy.** Clean diets comprised of food as close as possible to their original form (unprocessed) will help reduce and ease daily feelings of depression and anxiety.

STRESS AND YOUR DIET

Stress can be acute or chronic, both of which can affect your diet. **Acute stress refers to stress we experience for a brief amount of time.** Examples include preparing for a big presentation, or being stuck in traffic and running late for a meeting. Acute stress will likely increase your drive to eat even if you're not hungry. **Chronic stress refers to stress experienced continuously over an extended period, typically over months.** Chronic stress takes a significant toll on health and creates an inflammatory state associated with various chronic diseases, most notably obesity. Essential workers experience both of these types of stress at a higher rate than most.

STRESS IMPACTS THE BODY IN TWO SIGNIFICANT WAYS:

1. It affects our behaviors around food, driving what and how much we eat.
2. It creates the perfect scenario for fat storage and promotes an obesogenic state.

STRESS AND YOUR FOOD PREFERENCES

Have you ever noticed the types of food you crave when you feel stressed? You're much more likely to choose comforting foods or snacks, like pasta, cake, cookies, or ice cream. **What these foods have in common is that they're considered hyper-palatable** — high in calories, fat, and sugar and hard to turn down, especially when stressed.

Eating highly palatable foods leads to the release of dopamine, the feel-good hormone, which is desirable when you're in a state of stress. Over time, chronic stress may lead you to seek out that feeling more and more. However, you won't get the same reward from the same amount of those foods, leading you to consume more highly palatable foods to achieve that good feeling, which creates a vicious cycle. This cycle can create addictive or compulsive eating behaviors that become difficult to control.

Stress management may naturally help support a more nutritious diet as it's likely to reduce the instances when you may be driven to consume high-calorie or high-sugar foods. **Eating a diet full of color and variety will help ensure you are getting the nutrients you need to think clearly and feel your best.**

Let's begin with a simple top ten list. Again, if it seems overwhelming, start with just one! Live with it, experience how it makes you feel, and then decide whether to adopt it permanently into your life. Please do not get over-excited and do all of them at once. You cannot get the best read on how you feel when your body is overwhelmed by too many new experiences all at once.

Without further ado, here are my top ten rules for practicing self-care through your diet!

#1: GET ENOUGH WATER

Water, water, water. I have heard many schools of thought here, from drinking half your body weight in ounces daily to drinking until your urine is clear. For me, drinking half my body weight in ounces never worked because I was usually busy teaching and on the road all day, and this can put me in urgent positions, if you know what I mean. After a long day at work and realizing I am not at my magic number, I would guzzle water in the evening and then be up all night. Neither scenario was ideal for me, but if the ounce-to-body weight method works for you, do it!

Working in the professional athletics field for decades, I saw many trainers insist on monitoring an athlete's hydration levels for optimum performance and recovery by observing the color of their urine. This made sense to me, as your body usually does not lie; however, the one caveat to this is if you are on specific supplements, it could skew the color.

And if you're not an athlete, but rather are the average care worker whose daily drink of choice is coffee... you have nowhere to go but up! Finding yourself dehydrated as a busy essential worker can contribute to stiffness in the muscles, headaches, sluggish digestion, and stomach aches, so the busier you are, the more important it is to pay attention to your daily intake. Adding even two glasses of water a day and taking it from there can lead to big improvements. **Don't stress about a magic number; it's more important to listen to what your body is telling you.** Remember, we do not want to cause anxiety while trying to live a healthier life.

#2: PRIORITIZE PROTEIN

Protein is as important for busy caregivers as water. **Your body needs protein to build and repair bones, as well as make hormones and important enzymes needed for optimum performance.** That goes for busy people just as much as for athletes! Protein is used by the body to help create and support the energy levels needed to tackle extreme schedules and high-pressure situations. Physically active people also require more protein than sedentary people. Taking in adequate protein can help you feel fuller longer which can only help the essential worker who may not have time to take frequent breaks.

The same equations tend to come up in terms of protein intake as they do with hydration. Half your body weight in ounces of protein a day for one is daunting for someone like me, especially as a vegetarian. What's more important is servicing your particular needs. First, check to see if you are experiencing signs of low protein intake. These signs include craving protein, weakness, loss of muscle mass, hair loss, skin hair and nail problems, moodiness, getting sick often, and hunger, to name a few. If this sounds like you, start your day with a great protein shake and take it from there.

ACCORDING TO WEBMD, YOU CAN ALSO FOLLOW THESE SIMPLE GUIDELINES FOR PROTEIN INTAKE:

- Babies need about 10 grams a day.
- School-age kids need 19–34 grams a day.
- Teenage boys need up to 52 grams a day.
- Teenage girls need 46 grams a day.
- Adult men need about 56 grams a day.
- Adult women need about 46 grams a day (71 grams if pregnant or breastfeeding)

You should get at least 10 percent of your daily calories (but not more than 35 percent) from protein, according to the Institute of Medicine.

WAKE AND SHAKE

I usually start my day strong with a great shake. Here are a few inspiring recipes to start with:

COFFEE CREAM

1 cup your milk of choice

1 cup brewed black coffee, preferably chilled

1 scoop vanilla protein powder

Ice cubes

SPICY OAT

⅓ cup dry oats

1 scoop vanilla or chocolate protein powder

Sprinkle of ground cinnamon to taste

1½ cups water or milk of choice

Ice cubes

NUTTY NANA

1 frozen banana

2 cups milk of choice or water

Handful of almonds or walnuts

1 scoop protein powder

Ice cubes

MOCHA COFFEE MORNING

1 cup milk of choice

1 cup brewed black coffee, preferably chilled

1 scoop chocolate protein powder

1 teaspoon unsweetened cocoa powder

Ice cubes

RISE AND SHINE

1 peeled orange

2 cups milk of choice

1 scoop vanilla protein powder

Ice cubes

DREAMCICLE

1 frozen banana

½ cup vanilla or plain Greek yogurt

2 cups orange juice

1 scoop vanilla protein powder

Ice cubes

MINTMAZING

1 frozen banana

2 cups milk of choice or water

1 scoop chocolate protein powder

1 teaspoon unsweetened cocoa powder

1½–2 teaspoons peppermint extract

Ice cubes

BERRY BLAST

2 cups milk of choice or water

1 scoop vanilla protein powder

Handful of raspberries

Handful of strawberries (tops removed)

Handful of blueberries

Ice cubes

#3: CHOOSE NATURALLY COLORFUL FOODS

Colorful foods, namely fruits and vegetables, naturally contain most of the vitamins and antioxidants we need for a healthy, balanced diet. And, as a bonus, they have fewer calories so you're free to indulge and feel full. Having a diet that fulfills your daily allowances of vitamins and minerals reduces the need to waste money on expensive supplements, therefore simplifying your day planning. A diet complete with nutrient guidelines helps guard against cancer, heart disease, bone loss, skin problems, cholesterol issues, and many other diseases. You know the old saying: "An apple a day keeps the doctor away!"

When choosing fruits and vegetables, be adventurous! Try new and different ones often to avoid boredom and to have the best chance of fulfilling daily allowances. I often read suggestions when shopping that say to "eat the rainbow." I should mention again that when I say colorful, I mean all-natural foods, not artificial colors. When my sons were young, we removed all artificial colors from their diets and their moods, sleep, and behaviors at school improved. They still complain that on the days we took them to the candy store for a treat, they were only allowed to have white candies. We laugh, but it was all for their health, mood, and well-being.

#4: "PRONOUNCE EACH WORD"

It is tempting to succumb to easy, frozen meals — especially when you're tired at the end of a long, stressful day. That's fine every once in a while, but make that the exception, not the rule. **A good rule to live by is to read the label of anything you eat.** You should be able to pronounce every word in the ingredients list, avoiding high fructose corn syrup, artificial flavors and colors, artificial sweeteners, preservatives, and more. You owe it to your body to make fresh, simple, clean food choices. Eating is about nourishment, and when your eating becomes excessive or highly processed, you will not feel as good, will have low energy and will set yourself up for illness in the future.

#5: SHOP THE PERIMETER OF THE STORE

The perimeter of your average grocery store is where most perishable foods are so that they can be more easily accessed when delivering and stocking the shelves. There will be times when you need condiments and baking supplies; however, if you keep to the outer aisles for most of your shopping, it'll be much easier to avoid processed, artificial food ending up in your basket.

#6: LISTEN TO YOUR BODY

Many of us eat quickly or else disengage when we are eating, missing the enjoyment and the taste of our food (and often not chewing enough). For the essential worker, absentmindedly eating while considering the next item on your to-do list, or reading over a new report, or quickly eating while on the way to your next assignment...well, no wonder you end up inattentive to your body's messages.

If you take time to be mindful when you are eating, chances are you will notice and be clearer about foods that may disagree with you. Also, when you are focused on eating, you tend to realize you are full quicker and avoid overeating. When large amounts of food are consumed in a single sitting, your stomach acid has a hard time breaking down all the food. This leads to bloating, gas, and discomfort because the food in the stomach starts to ferment. Remember, your body is 98.6 degrees; you would not leave large amounts of food unrefrigerated in that type of heat, would you? Imagine the chaos in your stomach.

FAD DIETS

This also applies to so called fad diets, nutrition plans that aim to help you achieve incredible results by focusing on (or eliminating completely) a few specific foods. If your body processes good healthy carbs and you feel energetic and great, then eat them! If you can eat dairy without issues, great! When you are in tune with your body and take time to feel it out, you will notice if you have an adverse reaction after eating nuts, say. **Listen to your body.** It *will* react, so you just need to notice when it does.

A recent study done by researchers from Weill Cornell Medical College in New York City, NY, found that the order in which different types of food are consumed has a significant impact on post-meal glucose and insulin levels in obese people. **They suggest eating vegetables first, followed by proteins and fats, and lastly, carbohydrates.** This order of eating can control blood sugar, aid digestion, and help with weight maintenance. So next time, skip the pre-meal bread and start with your salad. I also find it fascinating that the way you combine your food can decrease the rate of digestion and cause issues.

- Protein and starches combined should be avoided. Example: meat sandwiches and an American staple, steak, and potatoes.
- Protein and vegetables are the best combinations for digestion and nutritional absorption.
- Carbohydrates and vegetables pair well.
- Fruit should be eaten on its own, with vegetables, or before meals. They are the first to digest.
- Healthy fats are neutral and can accompany most foods.

#7: PLAN AND FOOD PREP

Busy lives, especially those like essential workers lead, leave us pressed for time. They get home from work late, get up early, ready to start all over again. This will make you more susceptible to making quick and poor food choices. **One of the best things you can do for yourself is food prepping.** Shop for food when you have time to make wise choices and go home on a day off and prepare all your planned meals. This type of decision-making is healthy and conscious, not to mention a time and money saver. This strategy could also help you lose weight. If you have healthy meals planned out ahead of time, you will more likely stick to those meals rather than grabbing fast food or a quick doughnut pick-me-up.

#8: NOTHING WHITE

When doing your planning and meal prep, try to avoid white foods, especially white bread. Instead, try whole-grain fresh bread. For white pasta, instead try whole grain pasta or the new variety of pasta made with beans (which are higher in protein, as a bonus). White sugars? Try fruits to sweeten your cooking and baking, or local honey and organic agave. For white salt, instead opt for unrefined salts that are higher in minerals — but do keep to dietary consumption guidelines with no more than a tablespoon a day! That number can easily fly off the charts with processed foods. (Another great option instead of salt is to be creative with different spices to add flavor to your foods.)

What about white potatoes, though? Actually, potatoes are high in nutrients...when they are consumed as close to their original form as possible, such as with a baked potato. It's when you start indulging in French fries and processed frozen potatoes that you run into trouble with higher sodium levels and lower naturally occurring vitamins and minerals. Instead, try a variety of vegetables to garnish your plates.

White animal fats — high in calories and low in nutrients — tend to wreak havoc on your cholesterol numbers. Instead of these high animal fats, choose lean meats, high-quality plant fats like avocados, olive oils, and low to non-fat dairy products.

As a final note, it's not that *all* **white foods are bad.** Foods like cauliflower, onions, garlic, turnips, coconut, white beans, fresh white fish, poultry, quality dairy products, and egg whites, to name a few, when prepared in their original form are perfectly healthy. They just happen to be white, so feel free to add them to your diet.

#9: DO NOT EAT CLOSE TO BEDTIME

I know the schedule of essential workers often leaves no choice on this topic, but being mindful about when during your day you eat your heaviest meals makes a big difference in overall health, well-being and meal satisfaction. **Your heaviest meals should correspond to when you need the most energy.** When coming home late, or close to bedtime, your energy needs are lower, meaning a clean, light snack is a much better choice.

Not only does eating close to bedtime encourage acid reflux, indigestion, and mess with blood sugar levels, it interferes with your body's processes to rest. Your body is getting ready to sleep, not digest food! When you eat too close to bedtime, your metabolism is slower as well, so this habit can lead to unwanted weight gain and restless sleep.

If you are too hungry to sleep and must have a bite, make smart decisions. The best choices do not include alcohol, heavy foods, anything with caffeine, foods high in sugar, very spicy foods, or very acidic foods. The best bedtime eating choices are milk, which is high in tryptophan. High-magnesium foods like bananas, and cherries which are naturally rich in melatonin, walnuts have a trinity of sleep support like omega 3 fatty acids, melatonin, and tryptophan.

#10: AVOID SUGAR

Proper sugar intake and management could be (and is) its own book. To avoid this, let's just look at information about how sugar can affect your body and in turn reduce your effectiveness at work. In terms of essential workers, it is important to keep your immune system healthy so you can be at work where people rely on you. Sugar can suppress the immune system, upset mineral balances, contribute to the reduction of your defenses against infectious disease, weaken your eyesight, increase cholesterol and affect blood pressure. And that's only the tip of the iceberg of negative effects and stresses sugar puts on your body.

Long story short, I cannot find one compelling reason to eat sugar. **Next time you're considering a sweet treat, think twice for the sake of your health, well-being and job performance and choose other snacks instead.** A great list to check out is "147 Reasons to Avoid Sugar" by Nancy Appleby, PhD. She shares all the research and reasons you will need to motivate you to make changes for your health. Find a reason that resonates with you as to why you should not eat sugar and write it on a post-it note to keep on your desk, refrigerator or in your car to keep you strong when you feel yourself starting to succumb.

TAKE THE FIRST STEP

A nutritious diet helps balance hormones related to appetite and weight regulation, which can lead to better dietary choices and eating a diet more in line with your caloric needs, even when you're feeling stressed. Turning to food to calm your anxiety is completely normal, but it should not be the only tool you rely on for stress management as it only provides a temporary dopamine release and doesn't address the root cause of your stress.

The goal of this chapter has been to reinforce commonsense ideas that you've likely heard a hundred times before, but which you likely *haven't* been putting into practice in your own life. Whether it's due to high stress, lack of available time or the struggles of an inconsistent schedule, these simple tips often go by the wayside when working as an essential caregiver. It's my hope that these tips plant the seedlings of ideas and inspire you to research more and find a better, easier nutritional plan for yourself that helps you feel better, lowers your stress, and lets you operate at your highest level.

Something which has always worked for me over the years is to do regular weight check-ins to avoid surprises. I usually do an elimination diet once a year. (An elimination diet is eating super clean for 3–10 days without dairy, gluten, citrus, eggs, shellfish, and even soy. These foods are the biggest allergen culprits.) I have found my body to be ever-changing, so what once was no problem to eat is now disagreeable with my body. Once you eat clean for a predetermined period, you then systematically add one food group back in at a time to your diet and tune in to how you feel and how your body reacts. If your body reacts, you may be causing inflammation and encouraging other health issues to bubble up to the surface. There are a lot of great websites and books to help further explain elimination diet procedures.

These days, diet books and weight loss gimmicks are a dime a dozen, and the industry earns 80 billion a year. You have no doubt heard of or participated in intermittent fasting, Mediterranean diets, keto, macros, weight watchers, Nutrisystem, vegan, vegetarian, carnivore, paleo, the list goes on and is dizzying. You must do your research and do what works for you, not what your friend did to lose 30 pounds. Everybody has a different constitution and circumstance.

Throughout my life and career, I have become a human guinea pig for my clients, trying everything so that I could advise them from a more knowledgeable place. This led me to trying the "master cleanse" after all the media said Beyoncé lost 25 pounds with it. On day two I was fine but my back hurt; a day later, I took a hot shower to soothe my back and clumps of hair fell out. That was it, no more master cleanse for me! What was allegedly great for Beyoncé was attacking me...which serves as a great example for the need to stay true to the signals your body sends, learn, and make smart choices.

CHAPTER 4

GOAL SETTING FOR EFFICIENCY & STRESS RELIEF

"Everything that you are is a result of everything you have thought."
— Buddha

"Far better is to dare mighty things, to win glorious triumphs, even though checkered by failure, than to take rank with those poor spires who neither enjoy much nor suffer much because they live in the gray twilight that knows not victory or defeat."
— Theodore Roosevelt

Setting personal goals is crucial to success and is one of the best ways to start off a self-care routine. Most people go through life on autopilot, letting things happen and adjusting on the fly. This leads to increased stress, a reduced sense of confidence and control of one's life, and dramatically reduces your chances of advancing your personal happiness.

Goal setting is even more important for busy essential workers. It is easy to get wrapped up in the hustle of work, spending day in and day out in an attitude of, "Just gotta get through today." We forget about ourselves, forget our needs and neglect our health. But when you create clear goals with purpose, you are more likely to be able to find time for peace and quiet, say no when you are overburdened, keep track of your priorities and stay present in the moment.

I like to tell my students to think this way: Imagine you were going to build your dream home. How would you go about it? Would you just wing it and see how it pans out? Or would you hire an architect, tell them your greatest desires and goals for the home, draw out plans, and meticulously go over them for months, planning every window, every room, and each detail as precisely as possible?

Most people would prefer not to live in a "wing it" style house. So why would you want to live in a "wing it" style life? **Your life is your greatest gift; you should want to plan things out to make it the best life you can.** Just setting yearly goals is a great way to lower stress and achieve the life you want to live. I know some people are afraid to goal set because they think, "What if I do not achieve what I set out to achieve?" I say, "So what?!" If that ends up being the case, you can redo your goals, adjusting them repeatedly as your life changes and circumstances change. Dare to be optimistic for yourself: what if you goal set and end up *over*-achieving on every goal? Now you have to restructure all your plans because you succeeded too much. What a horrible fate!

All it takes is to make a start, and there are specific ways to go about it. Many people think they can write their goals and forget about them, but that is not true, either. So, let us talk strategy.

STAY THE COURSE

Going about your days, weeks, months and years without a sense of personal direction can cause stress and lead to missed opportunities, confusion, and many other unsettling feelings. Take, for example, a parent looking to encourage their children. When supporting your kids, everything is goal-oriented. First, your kids go to lower school; they participate in sports and activities you plan for them to help them grow mentally, physically, and emotionally. Before long they're graduating college and the ever-present question looms: "What do you want to do with your life?" So you help them plan, write and send resumes, attend interviews, and explore every option they can. It just makes sense to approach the problem in that way, right?

So what happened to this approach as you got older? Odds are, life got in the way and you started to let things happen rather than planning for better things. Let's try to consciously get back to that place of planning, forward thinking and goal-focusing.

The first main thought I will present before I detail how to successfully set goals is simple: stay the course. Most people, even goal-setters, will quit in frustration before they achieve their dreams. There's a story I love to share that helps to keep me on track when I get down on the direction my life is going.

In 1950, Florence Chadwick swam the English Channel from France to England in 13 hours and 20 minutes, breaking the world record. The following year, she swam in the opposite direction setting another world record, for being the first woman to swim the Channel in both directions. Those facts are inspiring all on their own, but the lesson she learned in another challenging swim in California is even more compelling.

In 1952, Florence attempted to be the first woman to swim from Catalina Island to the California coast. The sea that morning was an ice bath, and the fog was so dense she could hardly see her support boats, much less the sharks that swam around her. Yet she struggled on, hour by hour, with millions watching her on television. Alongside Florence in a support boat was her mother/trainer encouraging her. They told her it was not much further, but all she could see was the fog.

Finally, after 15 hours and 55 minutes, Florence called it quits. They urged her not to quit—she had never quit before—but all the same, she asked to be pulled out. She signaled to the support boat and was pulled from the 48°F water...less than one mile from her goal. She later told a reporter, "Yes, I was cold. No, I was not too tired to go on. I was beaten by the fog. Look,

I am not making excuses for myself, but if I could have seen the land, I might have made it."

It was not fatigue or even the cold water that defeated Florence Chadwick; it was the fog. She was unable to see her goal. Two months later, she tried again. This time, despite the same fog, she swam with her faith intact and her goal clearly pictured in her mind. She knew somewhere behind that fog was land, and this time she made it.

Discouragement, frustration and defeat are part of the journey of life. When considering your life and goals, failure of some kind is inevitable; it comes down to how you deal with it. Will you rise above and stay the course walking the steppingstones or will they be seen as stumbling blocks demoralizing you and breaking your will? This can happen easily to those of us who work long days that are highly focused on others. Just because you cannot clearly see the finish line does not mean you need to give up your hope and plans — not unless you choose to do so.

I remember a story I read about elephant training. When elephants are babies, they are chained in place so they do not roam. They'll try and try to break free, until eventually their will is broken. When this happens, the elephants need only be tied by a tiny rope to stay in place, despite having strength enough to break free easily. Even if a fire breaks out, the roped-up elephants will stay rooted in one spot rather than try to escape. A broken will is the only defeat that matters, the only thing that stops you from trying again. Do not let that happen to you!

GETTING STARTED

First, envision what you want your life to look like. Visualization is incredibly powerful, as we've discussed. Athletes visualize scoring the winning goal or throwing that perfect pass in any sport. **Goals give you both long-term vision and short-term motivation.** When goal setting as an essential worker or caregiver, the key is to envision precisely what we want our life to look like in future years. Working backwards from that vision, we can create the life we are truly meant to live. Goal setting is a compelling way of motivating people, including yourself! You lead by example as a teacher, parent, peer, or friend, so when you have goals set for yourself, people around you will want the same.

LET'S START BY ASKING OURSELVES:

- Are you happy every day?
- Are you living your dreams?
- Are you experiencing your best life?
- What would you do with your life if you knew you could not fail?
- Is every day full of possibilities?
- Are you contributing to society?
- Are you living to please yourself?

If the answer to these questions is a hard "No," it is the perfect time to dig in, get excited and be your catalyst for change.

Think about your life with regards to possibilities, expectations, achievements, future abundance, purpose, fulfillment, and desires. Write all these things down, along with anything else you want. Remember: this isn't an exercise in what you think you *should* have or what you think you *can* achieve; write what you want, no matter how difficult you think it may be to accomplish it.

POSITIVE VS LIMITED MINDSETS

You have a choice in the way you think and direct your life. With a positive mindset, you can achieve so much more than you could with a limited mindset.

What's an example of a limited mindset? Let's consider some common examples of negative self-talk:

- "It will be too difficult."
- "It will take too long."
- "I do not deserve it."
- "It is going to be too risky."
- "That will cause family drama."
- "It is not my fault."
- "I cannot afford it."
- "I am too busy."
- "I am too scared."
- "I work too many hours."
- "I get home too late."
- "I can't."

Do any of these concepts sound familiar to you? Have you found yourself lost in the black hole of this limited thinking? I want to bring this type of thinking to your attention. You may think this way and not even realize it, but once you are aware, you can more easily change your habits. That is all this is, a habitual way of thinking, acting, reacting, and feeling. When we are clear on what we think, we can more easily see the parts of thinking that hold us back.

Instead, consider some new thinking patterns. When you catch yourself in the old way of thinking, stop, regroup, and flip the script to be more constructive, using positive self-talk such as:

- "Anything is possible."
- "I cannot fail when I plan and take action."
- "There is only now."
- "I live fully in the present."
- "I must follow my gut and what I feel."
- "Attachment is the greatest form of suffering."
- "Stay in service. What good is success if it is unshared?"

- "If I can conceive it, I can have it."
- "With patience, I will create results."
- "There is a bigger picture."

There is a great Buddhist saying: "If the problem is fixable, it is not worth worrying about. If the problem is unfixable, it is not worth worrying about." This simple statement gets me through a lot of trying times. You need to start with a clear vision to create your ideal life.

LET'S START WITH SOME STRAIGHTFORWARD QUESTIONS. CLOSE YOUR EYES AND CONSIDER:

- How do I want to feel when I come home from work?
- What parts of my job give me the most stress? Can I adjust them?
- How can I find time for self-care in the most trying of times?
- Where do you see yourself in five or ten years?

Open your eyes, grab a pen and paper, and begin brainstorming. Write as *much* as you possibly can about what you *truly* want in your life, as if nothing could stop you. You might not know this, but once you start putting your thoughts to paper, ideas will come out that will surprise you.

Getting everything down on paper first will let you home in on what is important later. Research has shown you will be 42% more likely to achieve your goals when you write them down rather than just thinking through them. Think BIG! Write down lofty goals; after all, what do you have to lose at this stage? Get crazy. If you see yourself as the next Oprah or a professional golfer, even if you have never golfed a day in your life, write it down! Do you want to be a nurse leader, retire early, become the happiest version of yourself? Write it *down*. This future is just for you, so be honest with yourself. A good friend of mine was asked to set a mindset for the day after the passing of her son and she was at a loss until she saw a sign in my home that said, "I intend to be happy!" She was struck by the simplicity of the statement and how big the meaning was.

WRITE DOWN ALL THAT YOU WANT

I won't trivialize it; even at this stage of the planning process, some people get stuck right away. Their whole life, they've just gone along doing things unplanned. Now that they're asked to plan for themselves, they just act baffled!

If this sounds like you, know that a perfect place to start when setting your goals for the life you want to live is by thinking about what your gifts are. **Becoming clear on the talents that make you who you are can help you see forward to how you can best attain your goals.** This is more challenging than it sounds, so I suggest you ask your family and friends for their opinions.

START BY ASKING THEM THE FOLLOWING QUESTIONS:

- What are my key strengths?
- What is most unique about me?
- What, if anything, is bothersome to you about me?
- What do you or others rely on me for?
- Please tell me something about myself that I do not already know.
- When am I most powerful?
- In what situation am I least powerful?
- When am I most inspired?
- If you could wish one thing for me in this next year, what would it be?

Ask three people all these questions and write down their answers. After interviewing your three people, write down a list of any patterns and common answers you saw and pay attention to which responses stood out to you and why.

NOW, WRITE OUT FIVE SUCCESSES YOU HAVE HAD. HOW CAN YOU DUPLICATE THEM?

1. _____

2. _____

3. _____

4. _____

5. _____

WRITE OUT FIVE FAILURES, THE BETTER TO LEARN FROM THEM TO NEVER DO THEM AGAIN.

1. _____

2. _____

3. _____

4. _____

5. _____

WRITE OUT ANYTHING YOU'VE CURRENTLY LEFT INCOMPLETE OR UNFINISHED.

_____

_____

_____

_____

_____

NARROWING IT DOWN

Now that you have your vision brainstormed, you are ready to start breaking things down so that you can focus on the most critical goals in your life.

Goals are set on several different levels. First, you create your "big picture" of what you want and decide what larger-scale goals you want to achieve. For example, say you want to retire at 40 years old. Now, work backwards, breaking this down into smaller targets you'll need to hit to reach your goals. To retire at 40 years old, you'll have to make X amount of money to sustain the lifestyle you have and/or want. To make that amount of money, you need to make X a year, which boils down to X a month saved. Finally, once you have your plan, begin to act on them daily. You *must* act on your daily goals, whether it's writing 20 emails daily, cold calling, setting meetings, researching...whatever it is, do something each day. That is what I meant when I mentioned you cannot just set a goal and forget about it, you must take action daily.

MAKING A COMMITMENT

Be specific with your goals. If you want to work less and travel more, where do you want to go and when? Who would you have to ask at work for extra time off? Can you work shifts for someone else and use their timeshare? Set a course, begin your journey, work backward, and achieve what you need to make it happen. These are the essentials of good, actionable goal setting.

Remember what I said before? You would never hire a builder to build your dream home and tell them, "Here are the nails, sheetrock, and wood; go build it!" No, you'd take a lot of time carefully planning every aspect of the home, from how many bedrooms and bathrooms to the layout, where the windows are, how big the kitchen is, setting the closets, and the roof's pitch until your plan is developed. Once all that's been done, the house of your dreams gets built. The same is true of your life!

SMART GOALS

Smart goal setting is a popular, user-friendly way to iron out your objectives. SMART is an acronym:

S = Specific

M = Measurable

A = Attainable

R = Realistic

T = Time Sensitive

So, for example:

S=Specific. Instead of saying, "I will run a half-marathon," say, "I will complete my first half-marathon on July 2, 2025."

M=Measurable. Instead of saying, "I will start saving more money," say, "I will save $10,000 by July 2, 2025.

A=Attainable. Instead of saying, "I will complete four years' worth of college in 6 months," say, "I will successfully complete college by September 2025."

R=Realistic. Instead of saying, "I will take a big hike this year," say, "I'm going to hike the North Rim of the Grand Canyon by December 2025 after training for six months."

T=Time Sensitive. Did you notice? Every goal listed for the previous four steps had specific timeframes attached. This time stamp can sometimes stifle people; they think if they do not achieve their goal by that date, they have failed. Not true! If you are taking action on your goals each day and setting goals according to the SMART rules, then adjusting the date is just one more step in achieving your aims.

ESTABLISH KEY POINTS

When goal setting, it can help to decide what is essential for you to achieve in your life. **These points help set apart what is important from what is irrelevant, distracting, or someone else's goal for you.** They motivate you, building up your self-confidence. It is also an excellent idea to post your goals, writing them down and pasting them around your home as gentle reminders of what you are working toward. This way, there is no chance you will lose ground and not take action. Plus, your brain will start to believe it as true and increase your likelihood of attaining your goal. You have heard you can do anything you set your mind to? *That* is goal setting.

HERE ARE SOME ADDITIONAL TIPS FOR WRITING POWERFUL GOALS:

- Always write goals in the first person and present tense, as though they have already been achieved.
- Use clear, specific words that demonstrate commitment.
- Our minds also like specific numbers, so include them in your goals whenever possible.

- Allow yourself to see pictures of your life as you dream it will be.
- Always write goals in the affirmative.
- Always include a timeline with each goal.

For this last one, feel free to "time travel" to the future if you need clarity to help you picture it perfectly. Focus on five domains: personal, health, career, spiritual, and financial.

WHAT IS YOUR 10-YEAR VISION?

Take action. You should write 20–50 things you can do. They can be small or large, easy things or difficult, things that can take you out of your comfort zone. For all the things you wrote down, ask yourself how you can take action each day to get them.

By breaking your goal setting down into 10-year, 5-year, and 1-year strategies, you organize your needs and get even more specific about what needs to be accomplished each year to reach the 10-year goal mark successfully.

WHAT IS YOUR 5-YEAR VISION?

Take action. You should write 20–50 things you can do. They can be small or large, easy things or difficult, things that can take you out of your comfort zone. For all the things you wrote down, ask yourself how you can take action each day to get them.

WHAT IS YOUR 1-YEAR VISION?

Take action. Write 20–50 things you can do. These can be small or large, But for all the things you wrote down, ask yourself how you can take action each day to get them.

MAKE SURE TO FOLLOW-UP

These are the keys to following up on any reasonable goal that you set for yourself:

- Accept total responsibility for everything that happens in your life.
- Revisit your goals often.
- Revise goals if necessary.
- Find a goal buddy and help each other stay on track.
- Share your goals with people you trust for accountability.
- Create visual reminders of your goals (i.e., vision boards).
- If you get off track, realize it...then forgive and restart.
- Move forward constantly.

As a final word, do not let failures along the way deter you from your success. Stay the course, especially when you encounter a setback. In this day and age of social media and everybody thinking they have the right to comment on your life, do not let naysayers distract you.

On my first day of school to become a massage therapist, the teacher asked each of us in the class what we wanted to do with our degree. Many people had beautiful, noble goals set for themselves. I said, "I want to work with professional athletes!" the room erupted with laughter. I could have let that get me down or change my trajectory, but instead, I used it as motivation. If I had listened to them, I would not have worked with seven professional teams and over 3,000 professional athletes to improve their lives and increase their longevity in their sport. If you encounter a defeat or roadblock, ask yourself, "Will I let this be a stumbling block or a steppingstone?"

CHAPTER 5
MEDITATION MADE EASY

"Today is the oldest you have ever been and the youngest you will ever be again."

— Eleanor Roosevelt

Guided meditation is the perfect choice for highly stressed essential workers who want to gain the benefits of meditation, yet lead a hectic life where clearing the mind is extremely difficult. Given the experiences caregivers go through during work, alongside the lingering negative effects that persist even when the workday is over and you are home safely, the opportunity to find a moment for quiet, peace and introspection is as valuable as it is difficult to obtain.

In my decades of teaching, I have encountered a lot of self-inflicted hesitation when it comes to meditation; so much so that I prefer to call this process "mindfulness" to avoid the unwarranted stigma the term has for some people. Living a mindful life is so much more than taking a moment here and there to meditate, of course; it also involves taking conscious care to support your physical health, your nutrition, among the many other areas already discussed. **Meditation is one more way to help support you in your day-to-day life, specifically targeting your mental and emotional well-being.**

Guided meditation is especially helpful for those unfamiliar with (or unpracticed at) self-meditation. A recorded voice leads this form of meditation (though if you are lucky, you may also find places that do live in-class sessions). Participants follow along with the speaker's instructions, allowing themselves to decouple from the stressful situations of their everyday life. I have created several scripts for you to use (beginning on page 70), and I will also discuss how to make your own custom scripts to utilize in your life, ones which are conducive to your personal struggles at home or on the job. There are several types of guided meditation, aimed at topics like stress reduction, better sleep, reducing anxiety, or just taking a short moment to calm a distracted mind that may be full of trauma and unable to relax and steady itself — all of which are great for the needs of essential workers.

MINDFULNESS AND MEDITATION

Practicing mindfulness, even for just 3 minutes a day, can help you to find clarity and serenity. Imagine standing on the edge of a peaceful lake and tossing rocks into it. With each rock, you are churning the water, causing muck to rise and clouding your vision of the bottom. Each rock disrupting the peaceful water represents the things that contribute (negatively) to your hectic, frantic, busy days. Living in this chaos long-term could cause you to make mistakes at work when the tension is highest — a significant concern, given that many essential workers (such as emergency room doctors and nurses, psychologists, service men and women, and fire fighters) need to be able to make decisions on the fly with the clearest thinking.

Stop and visualize what would happen if, standing alongside that lake, you took a moment and let the water calm. Sediment settles back to the bottom and the water clears, leaving a glass-like surface that gives you an accurate read of the lake's depth and texture. *This* is mindfulness: the creation of those serene, peaceful moments of clarity between the chaotic rocks in your day. Next time you think you are too busy to do a short mindfulness practice, that's precisely the time you need it the most! To perform at your best, help others to your full potential and lower your stress levels, nothing matters more than a clear head and a steady hand.

During most guided meditations, you will be taken on a journey that leads to you controlling the patterns of your breath. This breath control helps calm the mind and slow your respiration rate. The guided meditation's script will likely include a narrative element, meaning you will be told a story of your body: how to be inspired, directives to relax, positive reinforcement, and visualizations that take you to a blissful place in your mind. You will often be given mantras to help keep the level of "mind chatter" to a minimum. I will discuss more about mantras later (see page 69).

While guided meditation is simple to understand, it may not always be the easiest thing to put into practice. It will take a little time to see results and feel the way your life and mental health are improving; like anything else, training the mind requires time and consistency.

Think of your mind as a rocky, weed-filled mountain. The rocks scattered everywhere are your thoughts, experiences, and habits. Standing at the top of the mountain, you are able to see clear paths to roll rocks down. Each of these paths represents a habit, a well-worn groove in your way of thinking that lends itself naturally to repeat use.

When you want to create *new* habits, such as more positive thinking, you're attempting to roll a new rock down a new, uncharted rough path. As you can imagine, the rock will bounce; it won't move efficiently. However, as you roll more and more stones down the mountain in your new intended path, they will eventually wear down a groove in your mountain, rolling down with the same ease they showed on the old pathways. In time, the old tracks, which are bad habits, will start to grow their own weeds and cover over making it more challenging to move your new rocks down the old path.

This is more than just a visual metaphor — it's representative of how your brain works to create new ways of thinking and eliminate old habits. **Essentially, you are creating new neural pathways.** When you go through a situation in your life, your brain adjusts its neural pathways and sends information to your subconscious mind to use for the future. With conscious effort (through meditation, for example), you can reprogram your mind to eliminate old unpleasant experiences and replace them with the new happier thoughts you desire.

BUT I FEEL FINE! WHY DO I NEED MEDITATION?

You may think that you do not need meditation because you are not currently feeling overwhelmed by life. Have heard the story about putting a frog in a pot of water? If you try to put a frog into a pot of boiling water, it'll react and jump straight out again. But when you bring the water to a gradual boil, the frog will not jump out; instead, it will acclimate...and then boil to death. This is how we go about our lives, tuning out our stressors, and then wondering why we had a heart attack after the fact. I think every essential worker can relate to this story!

You can even use this analogy during your visualizations. We are trying to eliminate the habits of overworking, feeling inadequate, and not make time to care for yourself. During these guided meditations, the goal is to stay present and not become overwhelmed with thoughts of the past or worries about the future, all of which we do not have control over, and which cause increased stress and anxiety.

Guided meditation is also a great choice for beginners and busy people because everything is laid out for you. You do not have to worry about the structure of the practice or if you are doing it correctly. Guided meditation encompasses breathing work, visualization techniques, and relaxation for you — all you have to do is listen and follow along. Once the practice becomes routine, then you can consider doing your silent meditations using the mindfulness techniques you've learned. With the amount of strain caregivers are all too often under, guided meditation is perfect for them.

Proper meditation and mindfulness are proven to reduce stress and sometimes can even eradicate it for good. For most people, once they sit down, the mind chatter kicks in: the to-do lists form, they suddenly remember something they were supposed to do and start feeling guilty for not doing what they think they should be doing. This is especially true for essential care workers. This brain invasion is the old rock path, the old bad habits. The same techniques used for stress relief can be implemented for relaxation and to improve your sleep; it all depends on the script you use. For example, when trying to induce sleep, the idea is to soothe the listener into relaxation step by step. Guided meditation can include music, calm voices, and pleasant and peaceful visualizations to encourage you to unwind, put your day aside and prepare for the best sleep ever.

VISUALIZATION AND TIME MANAGEMENT

The study of visualization use has proven that our brain responds to visualized situations as though they were real experiences. **If we visualize a stressful situation, our brain and body respond as though it were really happening.** Likewise, when you visualize relaxation and a life less stressed, your brain does not realize the difference and calms down. Athletes use visualizations all the time, as do high-achieving people in every career you can think of. Next time you watch a downhill skiing competition on TV watch the athlete before they take off, they close their eyes, and you can actually see them visualizing the course in their minds eye so that the body is familiar with what will be happening in the next moment after take-off.

There is a saying that what you believe, you can achieve, and nowhere is that more evident than with proper visualization; this is one reason guided meditation works so well. Take ten minutes to search on the internet: you will see many lists of studies proving the effectiveness of visualization.* You can actually change your body by influencing these biological functions, triggering muscle firing, and more. This type of practice serves to motivate you by demonstrating that there is no end to what you can achieve.

* I recommend looking up my favorite study, *Mind Over Matter: Mental Training Increases Physical Strength* by Erin M. Shackell and Lionel G.

Even better, you can have great results with minimal commitment. You do not have to meditate for an hour a day; twenty, ten or even just five minutes can start making an enormous difference in the quality of your life. You just have to make the time for it in your life and let the practice do the rest.

When choosing your meditation time, try not to stick it in the middle of an already hectic time, like dinner or bed routines, or on a short lunch break. The best time to begin is in the morning or before sleep. I like to set my alarm ten minutes early, and instead of going back to sleep I breathe and use my mantras. You can just as easily hook up your recordings and enjoy a less stressful wake-up with positive reinforcement to visualize the perfect day at work.

The way to enjoy the most success is to find the same time each day to do it; you can even put it in your daily calendar. As a practice example, I would like you to take ten deep breaths before each meal, or carve three minutes before taking your break at work to perform diaphragmatic breathing, or count to ten before losing your cool on the job. These techniques are not guided meditation in and of themselves, but they represent good mindfulness practices that will lead you toward better habits and a sounder life.

SETTING THE SCENE

Once you decide you are going to give guided meditation a try, there are a few things to consider first:

- Turn off all devices, including phones, radio, and the TV. Use only the device you are listening to the meditation on.

- Put that listening device into airplane mode so you are not disrupted by incoming calls or emails.

- Determine how long your session will be.

- Choose the goal of your session, i.e., relaxation, stress reduction, quick breath recalibration, better health, just to be happy, etc.

- Find a comfortable place to sit or lie down, where nobody will interrupt you or else put a "Do Not Disturb" sign up.

MEDITATION TAKES PRACTICE

The guided meditation process can be uncomfortable initially, but as mentioned, it will get easier with practice. During this time, you will inevitably find your mind wandering off the voice you are listening to, and that is *okay*. When you realize your mind has wandered, that is not a moment for blame, but rather an opportunity for mindfulness. Do not be hard on yourself; simply notice the chatter, put it aside, and start listening and following the voice again. Some days, your mind will wander 20 times during a five-minute script; others, you'll stay more or less on track the whole time. These moments when your mind drifts are irrelevant, meaningless. **Meditation is not a competition.** This book is about you becoming a better version of yourself so you can better care for others — not about becoming a "champion meditator."

Many meditations will use mantras to help you stay on track. **Mantras are words or sounds repeated to aid with concentration in meditation.** If you have ever taken a yoga class, you may have experienced the use of the word OM. That is a mantra. Mantras are great and easy to use; you can use any word you like that evokes a sense of peace in your brain, is not too descriptive, and does not stimulate a memory.

One way to figure out a mantra for yourself is to think about a current obstacle in your life. Do you feel you are overweight? Want to make more money or want a better job? Pick one and flip the thinking around into a positive thought. "I am healthy and happy and stay the perfect weight." "The manager at work sought me out to lead the team." "I am abundant and have abundant money." The idea is to leave out negative chatter. If you are constantly thinking, "I am overweight," it means you are constantly visualizing yourself at a point in your life that makes you unhappy. Remember how powerful visualization is — you are subconsciously creating a self-fulfilling prophecy.

ANOTHER WAY OF USING MANTRAS IS WITH A SINGLE WORD. FOR EXAMPLE:

- "Pretty"
- "Kind"
- "Accepted"
- "Accomplished"
- "Rich"
- "Calm"
- "Fabulous"
- "Delicious"
- "Friends"
- "Glamorous"
- "Happy"
- "Lively"
- "Energetic"
- "Believe"
- "Confident"
- "Enthusiastic"

The key is that your mantra should go in the opposite direction from your negative beliefs.

SAMPLE MEDITATION SCRIPTS

Before we start writing our own scripts and seeing what goes into their construction, let's look at a few examples I've put together.

FIVE-MINUTE CALMING MEDITATION SCRIPT

Get into a comfortable position.
Begin to close your eyes.
Start to feel the rise and fall of your stomach with each breath.
Notice the cool air coming into your nose on the inhale and the warm air exiting on your exhale.
Inhale...exhale...inhale...exhale...inhale...exhale...

You are now going to control your breathing rate to calm the mind, soothe the body and relax.

Inhale for a count of four... *1...2...3...4...*
Hold your breath for a count of seven... *1...2...3...4...5...6...7...*
Control the exhale for a count of eight... *1...2...3...4...5...6...7...8...*
(Repeat this series ten times.)

Now take a big inhale and return to your regular rate of respiration.

Feel lightness, calm, and warmth, and start to wiggle your fingers and wiggle your toes to wake the body from its rest.
Slowly blink your eyes open and roll onto your right side into the fetal position.
Take three inhales and exhales.

Bring yourself up to a seated position, and you are ready to go about your day.

SCRIPT FOR RELAXATION AND TENSION RELIEF

Get into a comfortable position.
Take a deep breath.
Feel your body in contact with the earth below you. Notice if it is hard or soft, warm or cold.
Inhale...exhale...inhale...exhale...inhale...exhale...

Bring your attention to your toes. Squeeze them and then release them.
Inhale...exhale...inhale...exhale...inhale...exhale...

Now focus on your ankles...up to both calves...to the knees...bring healing heat and light to your lower legs.
Inhale...exhale...inhale...exhale...inhale...exhale...

Now move your awareness to your thighs, release tension, and feel their weight on the ground.
Inhale...exhale...inhale...exhale...inhale...exhale...

If you have any interrupting thoughts, acknowledge them and release them.

Feel your hips on the ground and relax.

Think in your mind on every inhale *(RE-)* and on every exhale *(-LAX)*.

Inhale...exhale...inhale...exhale...inhale...exhale...

Move up to your back and notice any tension or spots that chronically give you trouble.

Start to breathe in extra deep, pausing at the top of your inhale and fully depress the abdominals to flush out the stale air.

Inhale...pause...exhale...inhale...pause....exhale...inhale...pause....exhale...

Bring a lot of *LAX* to the back and healing energy from the ground to your back, the structure that supports you each day.

Now move to your chest, shoulders, and arms taking time to let them melt into the floor on every exhale.

Feel your palms fill with heaviness and heat on every exhale.

Let the world's worries float away and roll off the shoulders, unburdening them.

Inhale...exhale...inhale...exhale...inhale...exhale...

Feel your throat and neck.

Notice your head heavy on the floor.

Notice the feeling of the hair on your head.

Your scalp starts to tingle, relax each muscle in your face and release the weight of worry off your face.

Inhale...exhale...inhale...exhale...inhale...exhale...

Take the next 2 minutes to enjoy the silence and the unique feeling of weightlessness and relaxation.

(Pause for 2 minutes.)

Start to come back to earth and take an extra deep cleansing breath and an enormous sighing exhale.

Wiggle your fingers, wiggle your toes, blink your eyes open, and take notice of how you feel.

GUIDED MEDITATION SCRIPT FOR STRESS RELIEF

Start in a comfortable position.

Let your arms rest by your side, palms facing up in a neutral position.

Gently close your eyes.

Start to take long, deep breaths in through your nose, feel your belly rise, and hold your breath for a moment.

Feel the tension build at the top of the inhale.

When you feel ready, exhale powerfully, and release it all.

Take long, deep breaths in through your nose, feeling your belly rise, and for a moment, hold your breath.

Feel the tension build at the top of the inhale.

When you feel ready, exhale powerfully, and release it all.

One more time, take long, deep breaths in through your nose, feeling your belly rise and hold your breath for a moment.

Feel the tension build at the top of the inhale.

When you feel ready, exhale powerfully, and release it all.

Feel the stress leaving your body.

Return to the regular rate of breath.

If your mind wanders, bring your attention back to the rise and fall of the belly with every inhale and exhale.

Inhale...exhale...inhale...exhale...inhale...exhale...

WRITING YOUR OWN GUIDED MEDITATION

Let's start by writing a series of clear, short, positive statements about you. These will help dissolve old unwanted beliefs and replace them with new habits of thinking.

WRITE TEN POSITIVE STATEMENTS:

1. _____

2. _____

3. _____

4. _____

5. _____

6. _____

7. _____

8. _____

9. _____

10. _____

From short statements like these, you can develop a guided meditation script all your own. We'll want to start each script by systematically relaxing our bodies. Usually, guides will begin with your feet and work their way up your body. For example, start with:

> Take a deep breath in and out through your nose and deep into your belly. Feel the rise and fall of the stomach and see the stale air exiting your body. You are feeling lighter and more relaxed.

> Start to become aware of your feet. They are relaxed and warm, and you can feel each toe. Finish this for your lower body.

Now, insert one of the positive affirmations from your list above. Next, systematically relax your upper body. For example:

Feel your shoulders come to rest on the ground with every exhale. *Inhale...exhale...inhale...exhale...inhale...exhale...*And bring your awareness to your hands. They feel heavy and warm...

Here, you might insert another affirmation here from the above list before continuing up your body.

Relax your neck and head, relax your mouth. *Inhale...exhale...inhale...exhale...inhale...exhale...*And relax the eyes in their sockets and give them soothing warmth. Relax every muscle on your face with every exhale. *Inhale...exhale...inhale...exhale...inhale...exhale...*

You can insert another affirmation here from your list. Finally, you'll want to close the meditation and bring yourself gently out of things by waking up the body, like this:

Start to take deeper breaths now and come back into your head and body, wiggle your toes.... wiggle your fingers.... take three more breaths. *Inhale...exhale...inhale...exhale...inhale...exhale...*

And start to blink your eyes open, notice your surroundings, notice how you feel!

There is no wrong way to write a script as long as it evokes good feelings. If you do not like the sound of your voice, ask a friend to record it for you. Record it on your phone or through a voice memo application on your computer. I prefer the phone because likely the phone is with you all the time, making it easier to fit meditation into your life. Speak slowly and softly in a calm voice, taking pauses between directions. Do not talk too close to the mic, as it can add distracting feedback or audio issues that can take you out of a meditation. Listen to your scripts as often as they prove helpful.

GIVE YOURSELF TIME TO SLOW YOUR DAY

Let's take a look at another script, this one focused on taking a moment to be present, to commit to slowing down. By doing this, you are sending messages to your body and brain that it is okay to slow down, that it is okay to release the stress. Nobody needs you right now; you are doing something by taking personal care of yourself.

Focus on your eyes in their sockets. How do they feel? Can you relax your brow more? Can you relax your eyelids more? Can you imagine your eyes warm and stress-free? Feel how your head hits the floor and be sure it is heavy on the ground with a tension-free neck.
Inhale...exhale...inhale...exhale...inhale...exhale...

Start to feel the cool air moving into your nose on the inhale and the warm air moving out on the exhale, taking all your day's stress.
Inhale...exhale...inhale...exhale...inhale...exhale...

On your inhales, think *LET*...on your exhale, think *GO*...
Inhale...exhale...inhale...exhale...inhale...exhale...

Bring your attention to your ears and tune in to all the sounds surrounding you. No sound is agitating. They are all soothing as they all add healing vibrations to your body.
Move your focus to your neck, and *inhale* LET...*exhale* GO.....
Inhale...exhale...inhale...exhale...inhale...exhale...

Notice how your head is feeling, full of vibration and warmth.
Bring your attention to your shoulders, arms, and hands. Feel how they are engaged to the ground, palms face up, *inhale deeply* LET...*exhale fully* GO...and send all the excess stress into your hands, filling them with the heaviness of your burdens and roll off and away.
Inhale...exhale...inhale...exhale...inhale...exhale...

Good. Your awareness travels now to your chest and back. Think about the weight going into your floor and through the floor. You are light and lifted, having released unnecessary stress that has built up in this area. The shoulders hold the weight of the world. We now let the weight roll off into your hands, feeling free and light.

Inhale...LET....exhale...GO....inhale...LET....exhale...GO....inhale... LET....exhale...GO....

See if you can tune into your heartbeat and hear the sound of your lungs filling with nourishing oxygen. They expand and contract. Go deep inside your belly to all the organs in your body and the miracle of their functioning without one thought from you. Notice how your lower back is slightly off the floor.

Inhale...exhale...inhale...exhale...inhale...exhale...

Re-lease, re-lax.
Now focus on your hips and notice any sensation. They feel heavy on the floor, anchoring you to the present place. Allow your attention to drift down both legs, relaxing from your thighs to each toe. Send gratitude for the legs and their commitment to getting you where you need to go. *Re...lax.*

Inhale...exhale...inhale...exhale...inhale...exhale...

Eliminate stressful thoughts, know you can solve any and every situation that comes to you.

Inhale...exhale...inhale...exhale...inhale...exhale...

Feel your chest and belly rising and falling, and again feel the cool air passing through your nose and warm air exiting.
Take two extra deep breaths and notice how the rush of blood floods your body.

Inhale...exhale...inhale...exhale...

Now let's bring ourselves to your favorite place.

Choose a location that brings you joy: your home, the beach, the mountains, or bed. Using your memory, start to set the scene and surroundings around you. Is it bright or dark, warm or cold, sunny or moonlit? Add as much detail as you can. The name of your favorite place can even become your mantra, for example: Bermuda, Aspen, Italy, or Paris.

(Pause for 1 minute.)

Now, whenever stress overwhelms you, you pause, remember this happy, safe place, and take three deep breaths.

Whenever you think of this place, tension flows out of your body, and you feel the most intense sense of lightness and joy.

Walk through your happy place, notice each minute detail, and smile. Are there flowers, other people, or water? What sounds do you hear? What smells engulf your nose?

(Pause for 1 minute.)

Inhale...exhale...inhale...exhale...inhale...exhale...

Start to find your way back to your body now.

You can always revisit this place anytime you want.

Start to wiggle your fingers and wiggle your toes.

Inhale...exhale...inhale...exhale...

Deepen your breath and blink your eyes open.

Feel how refreshed and ready you feel to go about your day. Set your intention to stay open in this present feeling filled with possibility and purpose.

GUIDED MEDITATIONS FOR SLEEP

Going to sleep and getting back to sleep can be challenging for a care-giver who has seen stressful intensity throughout each day. Listen to this script in bed and fully commit to falling deeply into a long sleep. As with the other scripts, record yourself reading this script, save it on your phone so you always have it.

Lie in a comfortable, supported position in your bed, which will be conducive to less pain and the most comfort. Once you get back to a state of relaxation and release, you will get to sleep. You will sleep deeply, and you will wake up fully refreshed.

Inhale...RE...exhale...LAX...inhale...RE...exhale...LAX...inhale...RE... exhale...LAX....
Inhale...LET...exhale...GO...inhale...LET...exhale...GO...inhale...LET.... exhale...GO...

Your breathing relaxes you. There is nothing left to do now. Nothing needs your attention, just your body and breath, feel your eyes heavy and your body beginning to surrender to sleep.
(Pause for 1 minute.)
Slowly release your next breath.
Inhale...RE...exhale...LAX...inhale...RE...exhale...LAX...inhale...RE... exhale...LAX....
Inhale...LET...exhale...GO...inhale...LET...exhale...GO...inhale...LET.... exhale...GO...

Let your breath flow as naturally as possible.
(Pause for 1 minute.)

Feel your shoulders relaxing, your legs letting go.... You are still.... Your feet are warm and cozy...
Your arms are getting heavy, falling through the bed. Your whole body sinks deeply.
Sink...deeper...and deeper...and deeper...
Your whole body is warm, comfortable, and cozy from the top of your scalp to the tips of your toes.
LET...go...let...go...
Inhale...RE...exhale...LAX...inhale...RE...exhale...LAX...inhale...RE... exhale...LAX....

Inhale...LET...exhale...GO...inhale...LET...exhale...GO...inhale...LET.... exhale...GO...

Your eyelids are too heavy to open, and your eyes are too tired to focus. It feels so good to leave them shut...*relax.*
With every exhale, the tension, worry, and wakefulness flow out the toes and fingertips, away from your body. You can no longer hold on to it.
(Pause for 1 minute.)

Visualize the tension leaving and floating out of the room. Your body is very heavy and relaxed.
Inhale...RE...exhale...LAX...inhale...RE...exhale...LAX...inhale...RE... exhale...LAX....
Inhale...LET...exhale...GO...inhale...LET...exhale...GO...inhale...LET.... exhale...GO...

Now inhale, count 1, exhale, count 2, inhale, count 3, exhale, count 4, and so on.
Inhale (1)... Exhale (2)
Inhale (3)... Exhale (4)
Inhale (5)... Exhale (6)
Inhale...exhale...inhale...exhale...inhale...exhale...

Keep counting on your own. If you lose count, start over at 1.
Keep counting and focus on the numbers.
(Pause for 1 minute.)

Relax back to sleep.
Release the thoughts, and return to the numbers...you are so tired and ready to surrender.
Your mind drifts away...back to sleep... deep asleep... asleep...
Inhale (1)... Exhale (2)
Inhale (3)... Exhale (4)

Inhale (5)... Exhale (6)
Inhale...exhale...inhale...exhale...inhale...exhale...

Back to sleep...
Sleepy...
Losing count... too sleepy to count.
Inhale (1)... Exhale (2)
Inhale (3)... Exhale (4)
Inhale (5)... Exhale (6)
Inhale...exhale...inhale...exhale...inhale...exhale...

Sleepy...
Relax now... stop counting... sleep overtakes you.
Back to sleep.
Drifting...
Sinking...
Surrender...
You are coming to rest, *sinking... deeper... deeper... deeper.*
Dreaming...
Calm...
Total relaxation now... and allow yourself to drift off into a *deep, deep, deep sleep.*

If battling tension is the reason for your difficulty sleeping the following script is a great option for you.

Lying on your back, take a moment to make yourself as comfortable as possible.
Bring into your mind's eye your "I am" statement (for example, "I am strong" or "I am healthy.") Repeat it quietly to yourself three times. *(Pause.)*

As you settle in, bring awareness to the spaces between your body and the contact it makes with the floor beneath you. Soften your body and rest. Your body relaxed, lying on the floor.

Allow your awareness to follow the queues as I guide you from point to point within your body.

Move your awareness to your mouth. Become aware of your tongue. Lower jaw. The lower row of teeth. The upper row of teeth. Gums. Upper lip. Lower lip. Space between your lips. Both cheeks. Right ear. Left ear. Forehead. Both temples. Top of the head. Back of the head. Tip of the nose. Right nostril. The left nostril. Right eyelid. Left eyelid. Right eye. Left eye. Right eyebrow. Left eyebrow. Space between the eyebrows.

Now go to the right hand. The right-hand thumb. Second finger. Third finger. Fourth finger. Little finger. Palm of the hand. Back of the hand. Wrist. Forearm. Elbow. Upper arm. Shoulder. Right armpit. Ribs. Waist. Hip. Right thigh. Knee. Calf. Ankle. Heel. The sole of the foot. Top of the foot. Right big toe. Second toe. Third toe. Fourth toe. Little toe. Go to the left hand. The left-hand thumb. Second finger. Third finger. Fourth finger. Little finger. Palm of the hand. Back of the hand. Wrist. Forearm. Elbow. Upper arm. Shoulder. Left armpit.

Ribs. Waist. Hip. Left thigh. Knee. Calf. Ankle. Heel. The sole of the foot. Top of the foot. The left big toe. Second toe. Third toe. Fourth toe. Little toe. Groin. Right buttock. Left buttock. Lower back. Mid-back. Upper back. Right shoulder blade. Left shoulder blade. Back of the neck.

Back of the head. Right inner ear. Left inner ear. The roof of the mouth. Throat. Right collar bone. Left collar bone. Right chest. Left chest. Middle chest. Upper abdomen. Navel. Lower abdomen. Groin. Whole spine. The whole head. Right arm. Left arm. Both arms together. The entire right leg. The whole left leg. Both legs together. Whole front body. Whole back body. Be aware of the whole body.
(Pause.)

Now bring your awareness to your breath. Follow the wave of your breath without altering it. Picture your breath as a light flowing up and down your spinal column.

With your *inhale*...the light drifts from the tailbone to the crown of the head.

And with your *exhale*...it runs from the crown of the head back down to the tailbone. Stay with your breath as it flows up and down your spinal column.

(Pause.)

Now bring consciousness to the sensation of heat. Your right leg is warm. Your left leg is warm. Both arms are warm. Torso warm. The whole body is becoming hot.

(Pause.)

All at once, your body becomes cold. Legs cold. Arms cold. The torso is cold. The entire body is cold.

(Pause.)

Gently guide your awareness back to your physical body, lying on the earth in the now. Become aware of your breath. Your body is slowly breathing in and out. Without opening your eyes, become aware of your surroundings. The earth beneath you. As your awareness comes back, invite your breath to deepen.

When you feel ready, stretch your arms overhead, extend your legs, point your toes, and take a full-body stretch. Slowly roll over into the fetal position on your right side, a posture that resembles a newborn child or fertile seed. Continue *breathing... think... inhale... exhale... relax...* until you doze off.

NO-SCRIPT MINDFULNESS

If even these soothing practices seem too daunting for you, here are a few quick ideas that do not require any pre-recording or take a lot of time:

1. **Take 3–5 minutes to practice the diaphragmatic breathing you learned in Chapter 8.**

2. **Take 3–5 minutes to practice a mantra.** Choose a word you would like to focus on and set a timer for the available time. With your eyes closed in a comfortable posture, start silently repeating your word. Once you notice the mind chatter barging in, take a deep breath, acknowledge your thoughts and start your mantra over again.

3. **Use the same techniques as above, except with counting breaths.** Inhale silently count 1, exhale 2, inhale 3, exhale 4, and so on. There will be days you count to one hundred uninterrupted by extraneous thoughts, and other days you never pass 3. The number you reach is meaningless. What's important is staying the course!

4. **Practice 333 breathing.** Set your timer for whatever amount of time you have and inhale for a three count, hold the breath for a three count while trying to tune in to your heartbeat, then exhale for a count of three. This soothes the mind and brain and increases awareness of your surroundings. Counting the inhale, holding your breath, and exhaling will drown out the thoughts your mind tries to fill the silence with.

The purpose of this chapter (and guided meditation in general) is to motivate you to try simple techniques that improve your life. You do not have to set aside large chunks of time to calm down; you simply have to create consistency. Learning to consistently find time for yourself, even if it's only little bits here and there, is a great start to rearranging your priorities to include proper self-awareness and self-care. The next chapter will focus on the use of aromatherapy to amplify your meditation time or just improve your overall mood.

CHAPTER 6
PRACTICAL AROMATHERAPY

A roma oils have been a part of history for thousands of years, appearing in records from all major civilizations and with uses ranging from religious rituals, food flavoring, medicinal use, to perfumery and the masking of foul odors.

Before modern science, the properties and usages of different plants were discovered through trial and error and observation. Knowledge was passed on through generations as part of oral traditions, developing into herbal medicine and eventually, aromatherapy developed.

I first became interested in aromatherapy through my mother. My mother was a flavor chemist, developing the first formulas for the Crystal Light drink. From her, not only did I learn about shelf stabilization, formulation, flavors, and taste tests, but I also discovered the wonders of using oils for flavor and fragrance. She often brought home the purest essential oils to me, and I instantly fell in love.

Inspired by these childhood experiences, I started delving into healthy living from my college days to the present. To this day, essential oils are my first go-to for illness and any health-related issues.

CLINICAL AROMATHERAPY

Clinical aromatherapy is an alternative medicine category that can be useful in both inpatient and outpatient settings for symptom

management, including relief of pain, nausea, anxiety, depression, stress, and insomnia. Essential oils are used daily for their aromatic scents in perfumes, candles, essential oil plug-ins, scented aerosol sprays for the home, fabric softeners for clothes, hair shampoos, and spices to add flavor to food. These aromatic essential oils are growing in popularity, with the healthcare community needing to learn about essential oils, their benefits, and safety measures.

Aromatherapy also has a host of benefits relevant to self-care and the needs of essential workers, including:

1. Aromatherapy can alter brain waves and behavior.

2. Aromatherapy can reduce the perception of stress and decrease levels of cortisol.

3. Lavender aromatherapy has been shown to promote sleep.

4. Aromatherapy massage can be beneficial for anxiety and depression.

5. Massages done with aromatherapy provide more substantial and continuous relief from fatigue than massage alone.

> **Note:** Essential oils can be dangerous and toxic if mishandled; some are flammable, some cause skin dermatitis, several are phototoxic with a risk of a chemical burn or are poisonous if ingested. If you are considering essential oil usage, especially modalities that are applied directly to the skin, please do your proper research first! Additionally, perform small patch tests when first starting out.

AROMATHERAPY METHODS

Methods for administering essential oils include topicals, inhalants, oral and internal absorption. **For our purposes, we will only explore**

topical applications and inhalants, as these are the safest and most common for non-professionals. When essential oils in aromatherapy are inhaled, the olfactory, respiratory, and/or gastrointestinal systems are stimulated (depending on your chosen method of administration). When absorbed in the body via essential oil molecules, these molecules stimulate and release neurotransmitters like endorphins, activating the desired physiological result. The quickest delivery system is via the nose as inhalants, which can foster instantaneous changes in blood pressure, pulse rate, muscular tension, and blood flow — very useful on the fly during stressful situations, longs days, and low energy levels.

The mechanism works like this: Olfactory stimulation by aromatherapy travels via the nostrils to the olfactory bulbs. The stimulus then travels to the brain for processing, where the amygdala triggers an emotional response and the hippocampus part of the brain retrieves it and forms memories. The limbic system then interacts with the cerebral cortex, activating thoughts and feelings. The inhaled aromatherapy molecules finally travel to the upper and lower respiratory tracts, with molecules then traveling to pulmonary blood vessels, the bloodstream, and other organs and tissues.

The second common pathway is topically, such as by a massage, in which molecules are absorbed through the skin. [*] This can activate olfactory stimulation and triggers a mental and physiological response. The skin pathway's absorption of essential oils can reduce a person's perceived stress, enhance healing, and increase communication. The path is summarized as follows: molecules travel to the upper respiratory tract and then the lower respiratory tract, followed by the pulmonary blood vessels, the bloodstream, and organs and tissues.

Studies[†] have evaluated the effects of essential oils like lavender oil on sleep and found connections of decreased stress to improved sleep patterns. In the lavender group, not only was their sleep better, but participants also woke up more refreshed. By diffusing lavender, or a lavender blend that includes myrrh, frankincense, and bergamot, before and during your sleep,

---

[*] Jane Buckle, *Clinical Aromatherapy: Essential Oils in Healthcare*, 3rd ed., (St Louis: Elsevier, 2015), 15–36.
[†] Ibid.

you can gain the type of quality rest that reduces your stress. Another study shared information about how aromatherapy helped reduce stress and increase performance in the workplace using petitgrain essential oil. The study found that subjects who experienced inhalation through the diffusion of the oil increased work performance while feeling more relaxed. It showed an improvement in both the mental and emotional state by reducing stress levels and simultaneously increasing awareness.*

BASIC OILS AND THEIR USES

OILS QUICK REFERENCE CHART

OIL	SCENT	BEST FOR	MOOD EFFECT	WARNING
Lavender	Floral	Dry skin, relaxing	Soothing	None
Lemon	Citrus	Respiration, circulation	Invigorating	Avoid sun
Lemon grass	Citrus	Muscle aches, stress	Relaxing	Skin irritant
Mandarin	Sweet	Digestion, stress, insomnia	Stimulating	None
Melissa	Sharp, floral	Stress, respiration, hormone	Revitalizing	Skin irritant
Myrrh	Smoky	Respiration, menstrual issues	Stimulating	Avoid if pregnant

* Angela Smith Lillehei et al., "Effect of Inhaled Lavender and Sleep Hygiene on Self-Reported Sleep Issues: A Randomized Controlled Trial," *Journal of Alternative and Complementary Medicine 21*, no. 7, (July 2015), 430-8. https://doi.org 10.1089/ acm.2014.0327.

OIL	SCENT	BEST FOR	MOOD EFFECT	WARNING
Neroli	Floral	Stress, digestion, dry skin	Uplifting	None
Orange	Sweet	Respiration, oily skin	Calming	Avoid sun
Patchouli	Earthy	Aphrodisiac, skin damage	Soothing, sensual	None
Peppermint	Mint	Digestion, cooling, sore feet	Refreshing	Avoid if pregnant
Pine	Fresh	Skin damage, muscle aches	Stimulating	Skin irritant
Rose	Floral	Dry skin, anxiety	Uplifting	Avoid if pregnant
Rosemary	Floral	Digestion, pain relief	Invigorating	Avoid if pregnant or epileptic
Sandalwood	Woody	Respiratory infection	Relaxing, soothing	None
Sage	Camphor	Fever, joint pain	Astringent, cooling	Avoid if pregnant
Tea tree	Antiseptic	Respiratory, fungal, skin infections	Cleansing	Skin irritant
Thyme	Spicy	Appetite stimulant, infections	Antiseptic	Avoid if pregnant
Ylang ylang	Floral	Stress, depression	Calming	Skin irritant

LAVENDER ESSENTIAL OIL. One of the most common essential oils for relaxation is lavender. Lavender essential oil is a great choice if you find yourself experiencing stress, sleeplessness, and anxiety. It reconditions the nervous system by decreasing blood pressure and heart rate, thereby calming the nerves, soothing restlessness, and improving sleep.

ROSE ESSENTIAL OIL. Rose essential oil is for soothing emotions and headaches and balancing hormones. Rose supports the heart during high stress, grief, and depression.

YLANG YLANG ESSENTIAL OIL. Ylang ylang essential oil stimulates feelings of comfort and joy. It reduces heart rate, improves your mood, and helps aid relaxation. Inhaling ylang ylang can help release negative emotions, reduce stress, and may well become your go-to for anxiety and mild depression relief.

BERGAMOT ESSENTIAL OIL. Bergamot essential oil is produced from the peel of a citrus fruit. It is often used to improve energy, fight bacterial infections, and assist digestive health. Bergamot essential oil improves circulation and encourages hormonal secretions and digestive health. It is a good choice as an antidepressant aid due to its mood-enhancing qualities and energy.

GERMAN CHAMOMILE ESSENTIAL OIL. Chamomile promotes calm, reduces anxiety, and soothes the nervous system. It can also ease digestive tract inflammation and regulate mood and stress levels.

MELISSA ESSENTIAL OIL. Melissa, also known as lemon balm, has been used for hundreds of years due to its medicinal and uplifting qualities. Called the "elixir of life," melissa essential oil soothes the mind, increases immunity, and supports the nervous system.

JASMINE ESSENTIAL OIL. Jasmine essential oil is a remedy for anxiety, stress, insomnia, and depression. It is used to detox and clear the respiratory system. It also acts as a natural relaxant, has a stimulating effect on the brain, and elevates mood and energy levels.

CLARY SAGE ESSENTIAL OIL. Clary sage is effective in quieting stress and anxiety. This oil acts as an antidepressant by fostering comfort and inner peace. Clary sage is also known to act as a hormone balancer and aids with PMS issues.

NEROLI ESSENTIAL OIL. Neroli can be beneficial for many ailments, including anxiety relief, regulation of metabolism, releasing anger and irritability, and easing worry.

BASIL ESSENTIAL OIL. Basil essential oil reduces anxiety and enhances mood, calms the nervous system, fights fatigue, and reduces mental strain and depression. It is also a natural stimulant, fostering peace and clearness of mind.

CEDARWOOD ESSENTIAL OIL. Cedarwood oil is a warm, woody scent that is grounding and calming, promoting a great night's sleep.

VETIVER ESSENTIAL OIL. This grass has a rich, exotic aroma that is incredibly grounding for emotions and relaxing for the body.

TEA TREE ESSENTIAL OIL. Tea tree essential oil is an effective deterrent against various strains of bacteria, some of which have developed antibiotic resistance. The oil can also effectively help eradicate specific types of fungus. Tea tree oil helps to eliminate the virus that causes cold sores, the common cold, and the flu, and is even an effective treatment for dandruff.

EUCALYPTUS ESSENTIAL OIL. Eucalyptus essential oil can help treat symptoms like fever, body pains, and congestion.

SAGE ESSENTIAL OIL. Sage essential oil can aid with digestive, breathing, and menstrual problems.

MAKING YOUR OWN AROMATHERAPY KITS

Creating your own at-home aromatherapy kit is easier than you might think! The materials and equipment you'll need will depend on the delivery method you're intending to utilize, but in general:

INHALANTS

FOR INHALANTS, YOU WILL NEED:

- An aromatherapy inhalant case
- Cotton wick inserts
- Toppers
- High-quality essential oil

First, assemble your components and select an appropriate recipe (see pages 95–100 for some examples). Take the top off the inhalant case and place a cotton wick inside. Drop the oils onto the wick, close the inhalant case tightly and give it a good shake before placing the cap on.

To use your prepared inhalant, first open the cap and place the inhalant into your nostril while closing the opposite nostril. Take a big inhale; you should notice the effects quickly, be they calming, antiviral, stress reduction, or protection from germs.

SPRAYS

IF YOU'D PREFER TO USE A SPRAY, YOU WILL NEED THE FOLLOWING:

- High-quality essential oils
- 2–4 ounce glass spray bottle, preferably dark in color (to preserve the integrity of the oils)
- Witch hazel

First, assemble the appropriate equipment and select your preferred recipe (again, see pages 95–100 for some of my favorites). Mix the ingredients and shake gently the spray bottle gently.

To use, spray your mixture in the air, on linens, on your pillow, basically anywhere you'd like to smell nice. Enjoy!

DIFFUSERS

FOR DIFFUSERS, YOU WILL NEED THE FOLLOWING:

- Bowl
- Small funnel
- Small bottle or vase
- Bamboo reeds or skewers
- High-quality essential oils
- ¼ cup unscented carrier oil
- 3 tablespoons rubbing alcohol or witch hazel

First, assemble the equipment specified and select your recipe. Mix all the ingredients together in a bowl, then use a funnel to pour your mixture into your glass bottle or vase. Finally, insert the bamboo reeds.

To use, find an appropriate place for your aromatherapy sessions and flip the reeds every few days. Refill the glass bottle when all the oil evaporates.

SCRUBS

FOR SCRUBS, YOU WILL NEED THE FOLLOWING:

- Granulated sugar
- Fractionated coconut oil
- Essential oils
- Glass/plastic jars, preferably dark in color (to preserve the integrity of the oils)

First, assemble your equipment and select the aromatherapy recipe you'd like to use. Mix all the ingredients in your glass or plastic jar and give it a good shake.

Keep the jar to hand in your bath or shower for a luxurious, detoxing, stress-reducing body scrub.

MASSAGE OILS

TO PREPARE MASSAGE OILS, YOU WILL NEED THE FOLLOWING:

- Carrier oil
- Mixing pot
- High-quality essential oils
- Glass/plastic bottles (plastic is preferable)

First, assemble the ingredients called for in your preferred recipe (see pages 95–100). Mix together, then funnel into your prepared bottle. Give it a good shake.

To use, slather the oils generously on your body after a shower or anytime you need a mood boost. Breathe deeply and enjoy!

ESSENTIAL OIL RECIPES

In the following pages, I've included some of my personal favorite recipes for essential oil aromatherapy. **Please take these recipes as a guide, and do not be afraid to be creative and listen to your senses.** Try to feel how your body reacts to each scent and make necessary substitutions. No matter what research says, it will not soothe your discomfort if you do not like the smell of a particular oil.

ESSENTIAL WORKER FIRST AID KIT

For the essential worker on the job and on the go, essential oils can be used to enhance existing parts of a personal hygiene and first aid kit. Here are just a few of my favorite examples (along with my personal recipes!)

HAND SANITIZER

1 ounce aloe vera gel

7 drops black spruce oil

7 drops lavender oil

6 drops cedarwood oil

Make this blend in a 1-ounce bottle with a pop-up cap (sometimes called a flip-top).

MUSCLE TENSION AND HEADACHE INHALER

8 drops rosemary oil

3 drops black spruce oil

3 drops lavender oil

2 drops peppermint oil

BUG SPRAY

6 drops citronella oil

5 drops eucalyptus oil

5 drops peppermint oil

Fill a bottle with distilled water or witch hazel, then combine. Other widely used oils for repellency are catnip oil, clove oil, and geranium.

FIRST AID SPRAY FOR CUTS AND SCRAPES

5 drops lavender oil

5 drops tea tree oil

3 drops basil oil

BALANCING FACE MIST

2 tablespoons raw apple cider vinegar

5 drops lavender oil

5 drops chamomile oil

1 drop jojoba oil

1 cup distilled water

Prepare this in a 2-ounce spray bottle. Harsh cleansers and makeup removers are highly alkaline, making them dissolve grime and products from your face. However, they can also cause your skin's pH balance to become out of whack. A facial spray that's slightly acidic rebalances your pH and refreshes.

ROOM SPRAY

10 drops vanilla oil

10 drops lavender oil

1 tablespoon witch hazel

Prepare this non-toxic alternative in a 4-ounce spray bottle. Be creative here with whatever scent you like for your spaces. Most commercial/store-bought room sprays have dangerous chemicals that are known cancer causers. These chemicals can also disrupt the endocrine system and affect hormone levels.

CAR FRESHENER SPRAY

5 drops eucalyptus oil

5 drops peppermint oil

Distilled water to the top

Prepare this in a 1 ounce spray bottle.

RECIPES FOR YOUR DAILY NEEDS

The following recipes can be used as inhalants, linen sprays, diffusers, scrubs, or massage oils. For linen sprays, fill a container with witch hazel and water. For reed diffusers, fill a container with 80 percent water and 20 percent alcohol. When you are making scrubs, fill your jar with oil and a scrub material (such as salt or sugar). I personally do not measure the mix until it has the consistency I like. When making massage oils or body oils, top off the container with the carrier oil of your choice such as aloe, sweet almond, olive or jojoba.

ANXIETY RELIEF

5 drops lavender oil

2 drops roman chamomile

4 drops ylang ylang

4 drops lavender oil

3 drops cedarwood oil

3 drops frankincense oil

2 drops mandarin oil

2 drops lavender oil

2 drops vetiver oil

1 drop rose oil

2 drops of lavender oil

2 drops of geranium oil

1 drop roman chamomile oil

5 drops clary sage oil

2 drops ylang ylang

5 drops bergamot oil

3 drops frankincense oil

2 drops orange oil

2 drops lavender oil

STRESS RELIEF

5 drops geranium oil

10 drops lavender oil

5 drops rose oil

---

4 drops tea tree oil

2 drops lemon oil

3 drops lime oil

---

3 drops orange oil

5 drops clove oil

5 drops cedarwood oil

5 drops lemon oil

---

5 drops grapefruit oil

3 drops orange oils

2 drops lemon oil

1 drop bergamot oil

2 drops bergamot oil

---

2 drops frankincense oil

2 drops lemon oil

10 drops lavender oil

10 drops bergamot oil

10 drops frankincense oil

10 drops myrrh oil

SLEEP

8 drops lavender oil

---

5 drops lavender oil

4 drops cedarwood oil

2 drops eucalyptus oil

1 drop frankincense oil

---

2 drops lavender oil

3 drops chamomile oil

3 drops bergamot oil

---

4 drops lavender oil

2 drops peppermint oil

2 drops eucalyptus oil

1 drop lemon oil

---

2 drops ylang ylang oil

1 drop bergamot oil

1 drop roman chamomile oil

1 drop lavender oil

IMMUNITY BOOSTERS

1 drop cinnamon bark oil

1 drop clove oil

4 drops orange oil

---

1 drop rosemary oil

1 drop clove oil

1 drop eucalyptus oil

1 drop cinnamon oil

---

2 drops rosemary oil

2 drops lemon oil

2 drops lime oil

---

3 drops lemongrass oil

1 drop eucalyptus oil

1 drop basil oil

5 drops rosemary oil

---

3 drops lime oil

3 drops eucalyptus oil

2 drops peppermint oil

CREATING A SELF-CARE SPACE AT HOME

Having a designated space in your home to help you find your peace and tranquility is one of the most concrete ways to prove to yourself (and your brain) that you're taking anxiety and stress reduction seriously. **This does not mean you need an entire room to accomplish this goal—it can be as easy as blocking out a corner of a room.** What matters is that the space represents all things that induce calm. Consider adding a favorite chair where you might read a special book or take time to practice your mindfulness. Make this the chair where you unwind after your long day and decompress from the happenings of the week.

Ideally, the area should include calming colors. If you are not able to change the paint, consider hanging a poster with a place you'd love to go on vacation, or a bulletin board with pictures of your favorite people or quotes that inspire you. You can also assemble soothing-colored pillows or blankets around you.

While you're in this area, try to listen to your favorite music—anything that is relaxing and in alignment with your desire to find comfort. Whatever you choose to place here should have a favorable tactile component, such as soft surfaces, smooth fabrics, or cozy appeal. And, in keeping with all we learned here about smell, it can help to find a candle or use your essential oils in a diffuser while spending time here.

Make this area your "take five" space. I know; for the busy person, constantly abuzz with a dozen different tasks, even the thought of sitting in silence in a safe spot can be daunting. 'How can I find the time to listen to music and sip tea,' you think? That's why we start by simply taking five. Five minutes is all you need to shift your mood, increase your awareness of your immediate needs, and inspire clearer thinking. Be creative, be open to changing this area until it inspires the feelings you are looking for.

CHAPTER 7

SELF-CARE HACKS FOR ESSENTIAL WORKERS

The tips in this chapter are meant to inspire you to create a better life for yourself, one which reduces stress and anxiety and reinforces self-care. Some of these are straightforward ways to incorporate more self-care into your everyday life, simple complements to the lessons we've already explored so far. Others are a bit more involved, but which you may still want to explore to really bring your self-care to the next level.

PINPOINT THE PROBLEM

When you find yourself stressed by your work, personal life, or the cumulative effects of past trauma, it is best to step back and try to see things a bit more clearly. **Look for the causes behind the symptoms.** It's all too easy to get caught up in the narrative of "I am stressed," and think no more of it. You can just take a pill and carry on, right? But that's not healthy, and what's more, it does nothing to improve the situation. Recall our discussion about visualization and mantra: the more you tell yourself you're stressed — the more you accept that as your reality — the more it will turn into a self-perpetuating prophecy.

A better option (and the best way to care for yourself) is to pinpoint the stressor and make an informed decision about what

to do. If it is a person, do they need to be in your life? Maybe it's your job; even if you cannot leave your job outright, you can still try to understand the origins of your anxiety and employ tactics at the first indication of the onset of stress. **Taking control of your life and owning a negative situation can empower you.** This is the first step to building a solid foundation of emotional strength. Many years ago, I was told to go through the contacts on my phone and identify 5-10 people that I did not wish to communicate with anymore or the people who cause me the most stress. I was then instructed not to delete them, because if they called or texted, I would not be able to identify who they were and perhaps then get blindsided. Instead, rename them as "avoid" in front of their name, Avoid John Doe. This way if they contact you before you answer the call or read the text you are well prepared and can take ten deep breaths to prepare your body and mind. I thought this would be difficult and to my surprise I redesignated over 50 people.

STAY ACTIVE

Whether you try the yoga in this book or not, the fundamental idea is to be as active as possible and enjoy the endorphins your body is designed to release. When your life includes regular movement, you will become stronger, feel fit, increase your confidence, and enhance your life. Building exercise time into your day can be as easy as turning our "take 5" idea into a five-minute workout. Walk, bike, do 10 air squats before each meal, get up every hour and do 10 jumping jacks, the list goes on. Moving may not eradicate your stress all on its own, but it will help you feel calmer and increase your oxygenation, which may help you deal with the pressure more evenly.

CHANGE YOUR TUNE

Do you ever find yourself trapped in a negative thought loop? "I cannot change my problems;" "Things will never get better;" these and other similar thoughts will make your stress skyrocket and your mood worsen. When you find yourself in these types of places mentally, take notice of it. **Make**

it into a moment for mindfulness and change your thinking. Start by rearranging the sentence: "My life is getting better every day;" I feel great when I breathe deeply;" these small changes will significantly impact your feelings of control over your life. Remember, deciding to be more in the driver's seat of your life is essential, so base your new decisions on what makes *you* happy, not everybody else. I promise — everybody worth having in your life will be happier when you are happier.

BUILD A NETWORK

It's tough to go it alone, both at home and on the job. Finding friends or trusted coworkers for support, seeking community, and committing to spending more time around the people you love will uplift you and keep you from feeling adrift in your own stressful situations.

There's a fantastic report I once read that illustrates the importance of this person-to-person connection. We may all understand this better post-pandemic, but this should help you keep it in perspective.

THE GOOSE STORY

You've certainly seen geese flying along in their classic "V" formation, but have you ever wondered what science has discovered as to *why* they fly that way?

As each bird flaps its wings, it uplifts the bird immediately following. By flying in a "V" formation, the whole flock adds at least 71 percent greater flying range than if each bird flew on their own.

When a goose falls out of formation, it suddenly feels the drag and resistance of trying to go it alone and quickly gets back into formation to take advantage of the lifting power of the bird in front. When the head goose gets tired, it rotates back in the wing and another goose flies point. Geese even honk encouragement from behind to bolster those up front to keep up their speed.

People who share a common direction and sense of community can get where they are going more quickly and easily when traveling on the thrust of one another. If we can bring ourselves to have as much sense as a goose, we'll learn to stay in formation with those people who are headed the same way we are. It's just sensible to take turns doing demanding jobs, whether with people or with geese flying south.

Here's one I'll bet you didn't know: when a goose gets sick or is wounded and falls out of formation, two other geese fall out with that goose and follow it down to lend help and protection. They stay with the fallen goose until it is able to fly (or until it dies), and only then do they launch out on their own or with another formation to catch up with their group.

If we have the sense of a goose, we will stand by each other like that.*

* academictips.org/blogs/the-goose-story-teamwork-lesson/

We could go it alone, but people tend to be happier and stronger together. Find your clan and meet up regularly, whether it's to sit together and watch TV, start a book club to spark thinking and conversation, exercise together...anything goes. All it takes is making a start. Believe me, cultivating these connections will prove to be a huge stress reliever. There's a Swedish proverb: "When you share your pain, it gets cut in half. When you share your joy, it doubles." A great way to spend time with friends and improve your feelings is to find ways to help others. You can volunteer your time to good causes or help someone carry groceries to their car. Helping others is two-sided. They feel good, and you feel good too.

ME-TIME

Finding alone time is also significant to your mental and emotional health. This time can be used to think deeply, do your goal setting, clean your house, clear your mind, or just focus on something that brings you joy.

It can help to make a list of things to refer back to in these quiet moments. Try it: what are some things that bring you joy?

1. _____

2. _____

3. _____

4. _____

5. _____

The first time I was asked to do this exercise, I froze. I had become so enmeshed in being a wife, mother, caregiver, and business owner I'd lost any sense of the activities I once liked to do. If you cannot think of anything right away, take some time. Ideas will start bubble up and you will once again remember the things you loved to do for you (and no one else). Me-time is not selfish!

CHALLENGE YOURSELF

Try to grow and learn continuously. After graduation and finding our purpose, many forget what it's like to challenge ourselves. Find some challenges to add to your yearly goals, whether it's reading 15 books a year, learning Spanish, taking five online courses, or running a half marathon. These goals should excite you and keep your brain fit and strong.

WORK SMART, PLAY *NOW*

I often hear people say, "Work hard, play hard!" and I could not disagree more! Why should your life be years of grinding, stressing, and getting yourself sick just to have a few extra years of retirement? Your years in retirement are usually not your best years. **A better strategy is, "Work smarter, not harder!"** Start some mindfulness practices by carving out your me-time *now*, spending time with friends *now*, and doing the activities that bring you joy *now, use the good towels now.* Now is the only time you have; later is not guaranteed to anybody. So set your goals, plan your weeks, make your lists, and understand the most critical tasks to complete...so that you can better ditch the stuff that won't make a difference. You only have so much time in a day!

LEARN TO LET GO

Being positive is important, both in your thoughts and the words you speak to others. **But just as big a part of positivity is what you *don't* think, what you *don't* say.**

My refrigerator has a magnet that says, "Let go or get dragged." Letting go of what I want my life to be — by which I mean, the ideal life I see in my daydreams — and learning to embrace, not just tolerate, the wonderful life I have was a game changer for me. Here is a great story that gets at the heart of staying optimistic:

> When my brother and I were children, we spent a few weeks each summer in the countryside. Our childless uncle owned a big house there and didn't mind having children around, so of course our parents were happy to loan us out for a few days at a time.
>
> Our uncle was a geologist and loved to go on long walks to find stones to add to his collection at the university. More often than not, we followed him.

One day we left early and this time uncle had us bring backpacks. "You can help me carry the samples," he explained. Sure, why not? The whole day we walked around the countryside and every now and again our uncle would put stones in our bags. We were also a bit surprised to see him periodically taking some stones *out* from our bags, but we figured he had just found better samples than the ones we already had. And before long, we had so many stones in our backpacks we weren't thinking about much of anything besides the heavy weight on our backs.

When we reached the house in late afternoon, we were wiped out. The backpacks were so heavy that my brother and I both gave a big sigh of relief when we thumped them on the porch. Yet we couldn't help but notice our uncle's backpack was half-empty.

"Why did you give us so many stones?" we asked a bit crossly. After all, he was bigger; why shouldn't he carry more?

"I didn't," he replied cryptically. "You did."

He waited for a while before continuing. "You did not know it, but I made you go through a little attitude test today. You see, I listened to every word you said. And whenever you were complaining about anyone or anything, I added a stone to your bags. Whenever you talked about something with an attitude of gratitude and positive thinking, I took away a stone. Now, look at your backpacks."

We did. And in truth, they were almost bursting at their seams.

The moral of the story is pretty clear, I'd say. **Your negative thoughts are like stones which you carry in your mind, just like stones in a backpack.** The more negative thoughts you hold onto, the heavier your mind is. A positive thought, however, cancels a negative one. So, take a look at your bags and start paying attention to what you put in them. The answer might just surprise you.

Essential workers are prone to experiencing stressful situations virtually every day, exposed to some of the worst that this world has to offer in their mission to give help to those who need it the most. It's all too easy to hold onto the negative feelings that witnessing events like these can generate, carrying them home with you, into the next workday and beyond, until finally you forget why you're feeling so rundown in the first place. It might well be that some of the negative thoughts you're having aren't yours to begin with, and therefore aren't your burdens to bear. Letting go of these thoughts and feelings can work as a cleanse, taking a load off your mind and providing you a clean slate to refocus on the person who matters most — *you*.

POSITIVE JOURNALING

You will automatically feel better when you recognize the positive things in your life.

TRY IT FOR YOURSELF AND SEE! WRITE FIVE POSITIVES ABOUT YOUR LIFE RIGHT NOW.

1. _____

2. _____

3. _____

4. _____

5. _____

Now take it one step further. At the beginning of each day, write down one thing you are grateful for and one positive thing in your life. Keep a journal and read it back to yourself when the stress gets to be too much and you find yourself in a tailspin.

CHAPTER 8
YOGA ROUTINES FOR HOME & WORK

"You can't control the wind, but you can adjust the sails."
— Jimmy Dean

We all know what stress is. Let's face it, we're all a bit too familiar with stress in our modern daily lives. But what does stress actually do to your body?

Stress can manifest as physical symptoms such as headaches, upset stomach, high blood pressure, chest pain, and sleep if you are continuously under stress. Stress can also lead to emotional problems like depression, panic attacks, or other forms of anxiety and worry.

Initially, stress also stimulates the immune system, which you would think is a plus. However, this stimulation causes stress hormones over time that will weaken your immune system and reduce your body's response to foreign invaders. Chronic stress increases your susceptibility to viral illnesses like COVID-19, the flu, colds, and other infections. Pressure can also increase the time it takes you to recover from a disease or injury. Now it may be evident why adding yoga reduces muscle tension, help you sleep, and improve your immunity for the best self-care system.

On top of this, how you handle stress can take a massive toll on your body in the form of muscle tension and pain. Your central nervous system oversees your "fight or flight" response. The hypothalamus gets the ball rolling in your brain by perceiving a stressor. The hypothalamus tells your adrenal glands to release adrenaline and cortisol stress hormones. These hormones increase your heartbeat and send a rush of blood to the areas that need it most in an emergency, such as your muscles, heart, legs to flee and other vital organs. After the initial stress response, your body struggles to return to a stable state.

When your stress reactions are too robust and happen too often, your body will *remain* on high alert. The hypothalamus tells all systems to return to normal when the fear is gone, but that response will continue if the central nervous system fails to return to normal or if the stressor doesn't go away. In the world we live in today, constantly in contact with our jobs, social media, the increased demands of parenting, and tough jobs, we live in a world of slow drip cortisol.

If all that is not bad enough, your muscles tense up to guard themselves against injury when you are in stressful situations. Your muscles will release again once you relax; however, if you are constantly under any degree of stress, your muscles may never get the chance to relax. Tight muscles cause jaw pain, headaches, and back, neck, and shoulder pain. Over time, this will put your body in a harmful cycle leading to decreased exercise and increased pain medication usage for support.

FIVE SIMPLE YOGA MOVES TO HELP ALLEVIATE STRESS

These five yoga poses are designed to keep you sane in the toughest of situations, and they are user-friendly, can travel with you, and require no equipment. From breathing to simple moves, regardless of your fitness level, these essential yoga moves will help you eliminate the pressure and be more productive, happy, on the job, and successful.

#1: DIAPHRAGMATIC BREATHING

Diaphragmatic breathing is an excellent technique to instantly decompress and change your negative stimuli. When you shut down the fight or flight response, you are simultaneously activating the vagus nerve which prompts your body's relaxation response to return to rest and repose. This allows your body to decrease your heart rate back to normal, lessen overall muscle tension, and increase blood oxygenation. While all this is occurring and your relaxation system is being restored, the reactive part of the brain (the prefrontal cortex) is allowed to resume normal function. When the prefrontal cortex is operating appropriately, we are better able to regulate our thoughts and actions—therefore performing our jobs better.

TO BEGIN:

- Sit up tall or lie down comfortably.
- While learning, keep your hands on your belly so you are more in tune with belly breathing.
- Keep your chest still and feel the air move in and out through the nose and deep into your belly.
- Do this for at least 3 minutes.

#2: ARM UPS

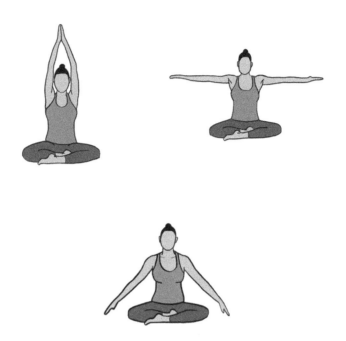

Arm ups is a yoga move that helps you tune into your rate of breathing and the specifics of diaphragmatic breathing. You claim your personal space and pump your breath. You can feel the pleasant effects of warming the entire body, especially the arms, and shoulders. An added benefit to this is upper body toning which is even said to help eliminate anger.

Do this for 1–3 minutes.

#3: SEATED TWISTS

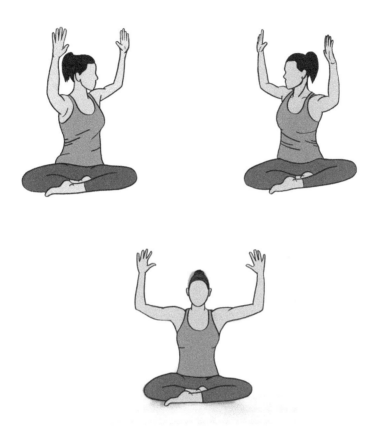

Yet another yoga move to help the body and lungs breathe more deeply, this move can also help tone the shoulders and arms with the added benefit of helping to align the spine and twist the body to improve its function.

Do these for 1–3 minutes, depending on your ability.

#4: OPPOSITE ARM OPPOSITE LEG

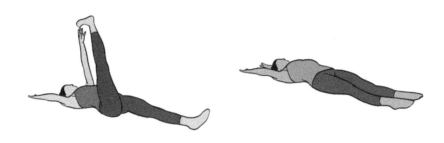

This move is a way to cultivate diaphragmatic breathing techniques and stretch the hamstrings simultaneously. It also helps warm the shoulders and feel the body get heated, which is perfect for getting you ready for your day.

Alternate touching the right hand to the left leg and vice versa. Do this move for 1–3 minutes.

#5: ROCK AND ROLLS

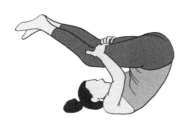
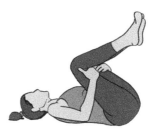

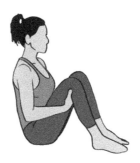

Top off your stress-busting routine with this simple and fun exercise. This movement is like being eight years old again. You will feel a nice massage effect on the entire spine (sometimes, I get self-inflicted spinal adjustments when doing this). This move also helps stimulate the nervous system, thereby restoring energy and vitality. If you do nothing else, do this move for 3 minutes a day.

Do this for 1–3 minutes.

TOP YOGA HOLDS TO RELEASE STRESS IN SPECIFIC AREAS

THE BACK

Back pain is the number one complaint I have heard over my decades of teaching. I've selected five stretches to open your back in all directions, elongate the spine, increase nerve and blood flow, and just plain old feel better! Relieving back pain and stretching the back involves opening surrounding areas, such as the hamstrings and hip flexors.

#1: SUPPORTED FISH

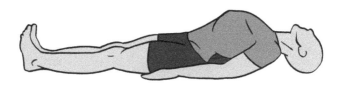

Supported fish is a fantastic pose to lengthen and decompress the spine. With deep breathing, you will begin to open the intercostal muscles, the muscles between the ribs. Opening the ribcage increases oxygenation and energy. If you have poor postural habits, this is a wise choice. This pose also opens the anterior spine from the throat, shoulders, and chest to the lower back. Put a block under your shoulder blades, ultimately, your head should rest on the floor or a second block and your hips are grounded, sink in.

Do this for 2–5 minutes.

#2: UP, ACROSS, UP, DOWN

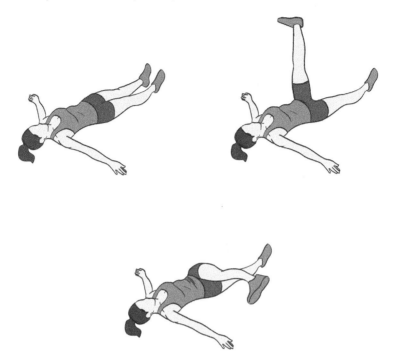

This yoga move does a lot to rejuvenate your body and increase energy. It helps squeeze out stale air in the bottom of the lungs, realigns the spine, and helps balance the brain. While doing this move, you will benefit from the increased flexibility in rotation of the spine, hips, IT band, chest, anterior deltoid, and calf.

Do this for 2–3 minutes, alternating legs.

#3: SPHINX

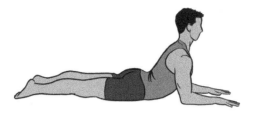

Sphinx is a counter pose to most of the slouching and forward bending we do throughout the day and is a more energizing pose with most of the same benefits as Supported Fish. This pose helps build functional strength in the shoulder girdle and arms and adds a lower abdominal stretch with hip flexor release.

Do this for 1–3 minutes.

#4: CHILD POSE

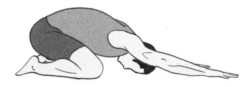

Seemingly everybody's favorite pose for its resting quality, Child Pose *does* have therapeutic benefits. It opens the side body, ribs, and lungs and releases the lower back. I like to have people rest their forehead on the floor or a block and gently rock the head from left to right, massaging and relieving stress in the face and brow.

Hold this pose for 10 breaths.

#5: HIP FLEXORS STRETCH

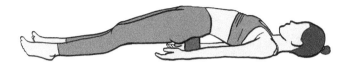

A hip flexors stretch on the blocks is one of the ultimate restorative postures. The beauty of this pose is that the block and gravity are doing all the work for you. The more you let go, the better. The block pushes the hips higher and sends the body into a mild extension. When you find a relaxing way to open the hip flexors, it tends to reposition the pelvis where it should be and take the load off the delicate low back. In addition, once the pelvis is realigned, you gain a bit of length in the hamstrings. This pose is especially critical for people who sit a lot. If the pose causes pain in the low back try moving the block a bit closer to your feet.

Relax into this pose for 3–5 minutes.

#6: LYING SPINAL TWISTS

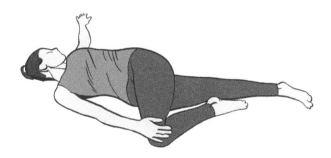

Lying spinal twists are the kingpin in realigning the spine and opening the ribs for deeper breathing. In addition, it helps increase rotation in the neck and stretch the anterior deltoid and chest. Do not cross your knees if it is too deep when beginning to practice this pose. Try all different angles of the arm with palm facing up until you find the best stretch for you.

Do this for 2 minutes in each direction.

#7: BANANA POSE

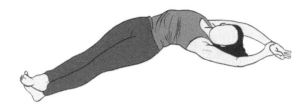

When people think of opening the body, they mainly think of flexion, extension, and rotation, often neglecting lateral stretches. The banana pose is the best lateral opener: it addresses the arm, shoulder, ribs, hips, and IT band. The deeper you inhale in this pose, the deeper your stretch will be. A more advanced version is to put a yoga block under your hips to add the hip flexor element to the suppleness.

Do this for 2–3 minutes in each direction.

#8: THREAD THE NEEDLE

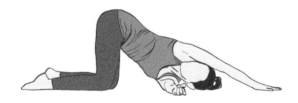

Thread the needle targets the latissimus dorsi which runs from the armpit area to the waist. In addition, it stretches the rotator cuff and trapezius with a bit of neck. The gentle spinal twist this movement incorporates is also a nice bonus!

Do this for 10 breaths on each side.

NECK AND SHOULDERS

It seems very intuitive when you think about what a stressed-out person looks like: tight shoulders with the shoulders tensed up into the ears. This can cause everything from neck pain, headaches, tingling in the arms and hands and decreased mobility in the hands. Often, I see asymmetrical eyes when someone has a tight neck and shoulders. Try these top poses to open the shoulders and neck. Most stretches in this set are great to do at work at your desk or while having lunch. Try to be careful when rolling your head to the back. If you feel pinching or pain, squeeze the shoulders into your ears when your chin is lifted to add support.

#1: NECK ROLLS

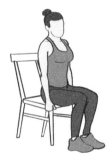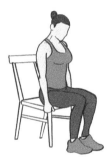

Follow the sequence pictured above. Do this for 3 rolls in each direction.

#2: CHICKEN WING STRETCH

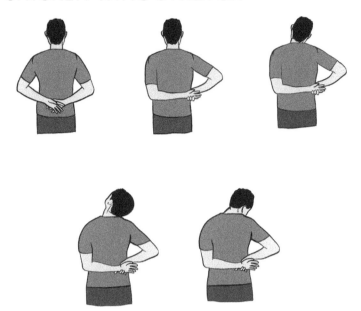

Follow the sequence pictured above. Do this for 2 minutes on each side.

#3: SHRUGS

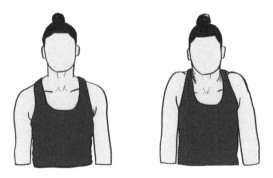

Follow the sequence pictured above. Do this for 30 seconds. Be sure to inhale into a tall spine and exhale into a deeper neck stretch.

#4: FORWARD FOLD

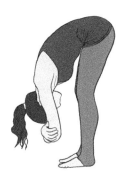

Perform the movement pictured above. Keep your eyes open for better balance and shake your head yes and no, to decompress the neck. Do this for 1 minute in each direction.

#5: CAT COW

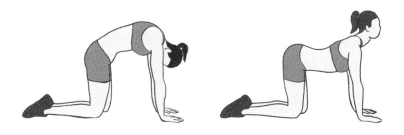

Follow the sequence pictured above. Do this for 1–2 minutes.

#6: FACE DOWN SHOULDER STRETCH

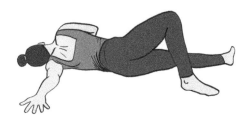

Perform the movement pictured above. Do this for 2–3 minutes on each side.

#7: FACE UP SHOULDER STRETCH

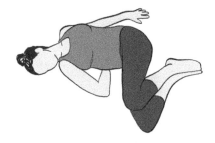

Perform the movement pictured above. Do this for 2–3 minutes on each side.

#8: FLOSSERS

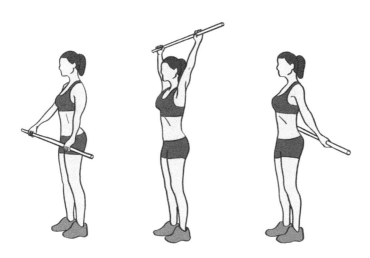

Follow the sequence pictured above. Using a yoga strap set your hands wide enough that you are able to keep your arms straight and get a great shoulder girdle stretch. Do this for 1 minute.

#9: PUPPY

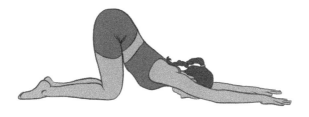

Perform the movement pictured above. Do this for 1 minute.

#10: EAGLE ARMS WITH VARIATIONS

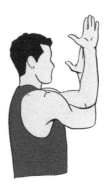

Perform the movement pictured above. Do this for 3 minutes.

HIPS

Hips are the most common place that your body stores stress. When you are stressed, traumatized, in fear, or harboring anxiety, you can be sure the hips will need time and care to recover. This area is more challenging to open due to the large, thick muscles, but you will reap great rewards with enough time and attention. An excellent tip is that when you are doing your hip stretches, focus on deep diaphragmatic breathing while *also* relaxing your jaw. If you tense your jaw and clamp your teeth, you will automatically translate that tension into the hips. Think of sprinters in the Olympics: if you watch closely, their lower jaws are hanging to decrease the hip tension and make their strides smoother and more efficient.

#1: DRAGON

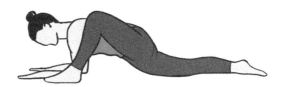

Assume the pose pictured above. Do this for 1 minute on each side.

#2: PIGEON

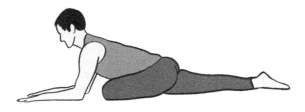

Assume the pose pictured above. Do this for 3 minutes on each side.

#3: EASY CROSS LEG LATERAL BEND

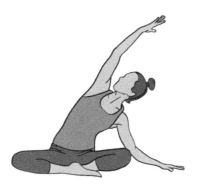

Assume the pose pictured above. Do this for 2 minutes each direction.

#4: HALF HAPPY BABY ON BLOCK

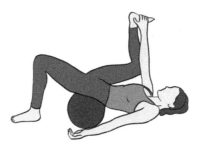

Assume the pose pictured above. Do this for 2 minutes on each side. If the picture above feels good then advance to lengthening your grounded leg to straight on the floor.

#5: HAPPY BABY

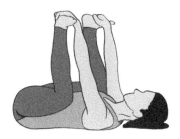

Assume the pose pictured above. Do this for 1 minute.

#6: RECLINING COBBLER

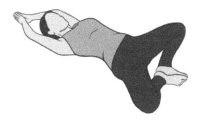

Assume the pose pictured above. Do this for 2 minutes.

#7: FROG

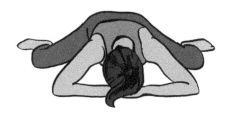

Assume the pose pictured above. Do this for 3–5 minutes.

#8: HERO

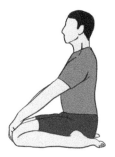

Assume the pose pictured above. Do this for 3–5 minutes.

SEATED STRETCHES

It's the common complaint of the modern workplace: hours on end, stuck sitting at our desks. While not always the case for the essential worker, odds are at some point in your day you will find yourself seated at a desk, taking a quick break or waiting for your next task. Sitting at our desks, coupled with the mental stressors of work, it is easy to build tension. Also, these static positions can tighten the anterior spine and chest and decrease the depth of breath. Here are some stretches you can do right at your seat to reinvigorate you and help you with the rest of your day. Do each stretch for 10 deep breaths.

#1: SEATED SIDE LEANS

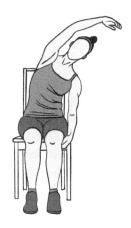

While sitting in your chair, inhale and lift your left arm up to the sky and over your head to the right. You should feel a great side and shoulder stretch. Remember to stretch the other way.

#2: HEATED EYES

Long hours of focus on paperwork, computer screens, or sitting with clients/
patients can cause tired, strained eyes.
While sitting, face your desk, take your
palms together and vigorously rub them
for about 30 seconds to create a lot of
heat. Once the palms are super-hot, rest
your elbows on your desk, cup the palms,
and rest the round orbital bone of the
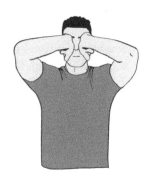
eyes in the hands *without* putting pressure on the eyeball. Take a few
breaths here and feel the healing heat penetrate your eyeball to the optic
nerve and brain. It is very relaxing.

#3: EYE MOVES

Once you complete the heated eyes procedure, keep the eyes resting in
the palms with the eyelids gently shut, do this series of eye movements.
Move your eyes straight up and down ten times, then from the left to
right ten times. Starting looking in the left upper corner, and perform a
diagonal move to the lower right corner ten times. Starting in the upper
right, perform a diagonal to the lower left corner ten times. Starting at
the 12:00 position, do five big circles right, then five big circles to the left.
Rest your eyes in the center for a few breaths.

This eye movement will strengthen your eye muscles and may even
improve your vision.

#4: SEATED TWISTS

While sitting in a chair, sit as tall and
straight as you can. To get the best rotation for your spine, you need to elongate.
If you slump, you will inhibit the depth
of the stretch. Bring your hands to the
right of the chair seat or armrest. Inhale,
get taller, exhale twist deeper for ten
breaths. Remember your neck. Turn your
chin over your right shoulder. Repeat on
the other side.

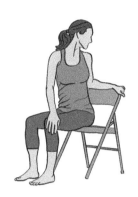

   This twist will realign the spine and wring out the organs and
lower lungs.

#5: LEG EXTENSIONS

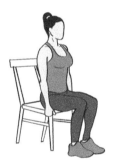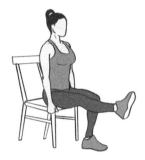

Sit tall in your chair, take a deep breath, and exhale. Straighten the right
leg and repeat ten times on each leg. This movement will loosen up the
legs, increase blood flood, aid lymph drainage, and help strengthen the
quadriceps.

#6: FOOT ROLLS

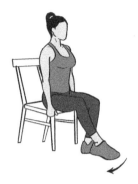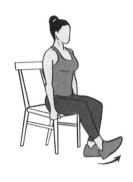

After you do your leg extensions, extend one leg and do ten ankle rolls in each direction. Next, do the same with the other leg. This move will help with circulation and stiffness.

#7: NECK ROLLS

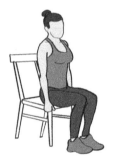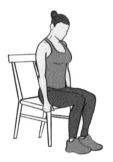

You may already do this innately, but I propose you institute this into your day several times. Do ten big, slow neck circles in each direction. If it hurts your neck to drop your head back, try doing forward half circles, chin to chest center, right ear to the right shoulder, chin to chest center, and left ear to the left shoulder. While circling your head, if you find a spot that feels particularly tight, hold the stretch there for three breaths and then continue.

#8: WRIST ROLLS

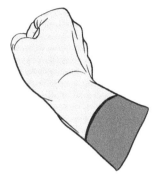 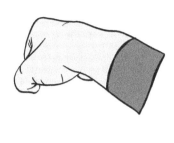

Like the ankle rolls, you need to keep your hands open, too. When you work with your hands a lot, you have a higher risk of developing carpal tunnel syndrome, which can be very painful and prevent you from doing your job. Sit back in your chair, rest your arm on the armrest, and start ten wrist circles in each direction with a gentle fist. Remember to do the same on the other side.

#9: HAND SQUEEZES

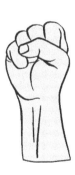 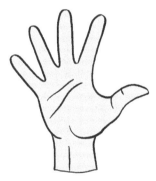

Even more critical than wrist rolls are hand squeezes. Starting with a fist, squeeze it very hard then open your fingers and spread them apart as far as possible. This will open the palm and the fascia in the hand and between the fingers. Do it ten times. Sometimes I take my opposite hand's pointer and thumb and gently stretch each finger apart a little further. You will feel instantly better.

#10: SEATED PIGEON

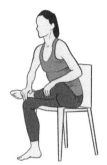

Seated pigeon is meant to target tight hips and back pain. Sitting in your chair, cross your right outer shin across the left thigh in a figure 4 position. For some, this alone is challenging. That only means you must be consistent with it. If it is difficult, stay there. If you can, round your back over your right shin and drop your head. Doing this pose will wake up your back and increase blood flow. Take caution when placing your shin across the thigh. If you are tight, do not yank it on; this will only stress the knee. If that is the case for you, cross your leg, fold, and in time with practice, you will get there. Remember the other side.

#11: SLUMPS

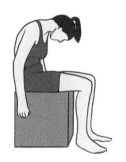

Just as it sounds, push your chair away from your desk and slump the head, chest, and belly over your thighs for ten deep breaths. This pose gives your back muscles a break and opens the posterior shoulders. Be sure to roll up slowly so you do not get dizzy.

#12: DEEP BREATHING

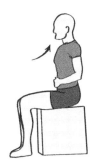 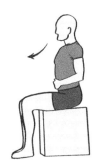

Every hour or two, to stave off anxiety before it happens, sit back in your chair with a tall back and relaxed shoulders and take ten deep breaths in and out through the nose. It is a great idea to put a note where you will see it or set an alarm reminder on your phone to execute this several times a day. I bet as you are now, you go through each day without a great deep cleansing breath. When you perform this, you will instantly tune back into your body and surroundings and feel the body vibrate with life.

10-MINUTE NO-EQUIPMENT ROUTINES

If you do not have time to go to the gym, don't beat yourself up. You can have a meaningful workout without a gym, a trainer, or any equipment. **You just need to motivate yourself.**

I know that's not as easy as it sounds. After a long day, the last thing you want to consider is a workout. I propose to you, for your health and well-being, that you do a 10-minute exercise. If time permits, I guarantee you will feel better, see improvements, and be motivated to stretch it to 15–20 minutes occasionally. You may feel like you're too tired to do it, but after you are done, you will never regret it.

I am giving you two concise workouts. **Give yourself the gift of better muscle tone, increased circulation, and a healthy heart.** Start by doing each move for 30 seconds, one time through. In time and with practice, you can do each move 30–120 seconds, 1–2 times through. Put a smile on your face and trick your brain into thinking it is having fun. It sounds funny, but it works!

UPPER BODY NO-EQUIPMENT WORKOUT

EXERCISE	NOTES
Push-Ups	Knees up or down
Plank Hold	
Plank Alternate Shoulder Tap	In plank, take the right hand and tap the left shoulder, replace left-hand taps right shoulder
Triceps Dips	Hands on a bench or a firm, sturdy chair, face away from the bench, palms flat, bend the elbows and dip the body up and down
Down Dog Push-Ups	In down dog, bend elbows out left to right and lower the top of your head as close to the ground as possible and straighten the arms

EXERCISE	NOTES
Fake Jump Ropes	Jump rope movement without a jump rope
Biceps Curls	Palms facing forward, elbows close to waist
Hammer Curls	Palms face each other, elbows close to the waist
Alternate Shoulder Press	Palms facing forward
Forearm Plank Hold	
Down Dog Walks	Start in down dog, walk your hands towards your feet, and then back to down dog
Cross-Body Punches	Hold fist like a boxer, alternating punch right arm across your body palm facing down
Jumping Jacks	
Roll-Ups	Starting on your back, arms crossed at your chest, slowly roll up to seated, slowly roll down to your back

LOWER BODY NO-EQUIPMENT WORKOUT

EXERCISE	NOTES
Air Squats Flat Feet	Regular squat move, track knees straight ahead
Plie Squat	Feet wide apart, bend knees until thighs are parallel to the floor and straighten, track knees over the second toe
Front Lunge	Right leg steps forward, lower left knee to the floor, step back to standing, alternate legs
Back Lunge	Right leg steps backward, lower right knee to the floor, step back to standing, alternate legs

EXERCISE	NOTES
Side Lunge	Step right leg laterally out to the right, bending right knee deeply, left-hand touches right foot, step back to standing, alternate legs
Standing One Leg Abduction	Standing, hands on hips, flex the right foot, lift right leg out to the side, pause, and lower back down, repeat standing one leg abduction on the other side
Jumping Jacks	
Cross Body Kick	Stand with arms extended out at shoulder height, palms facing the floor, kick right straight leg with a flexed foot across the body as close to left hand as possible, alternate legs
Standing Calf Raises	Stand with feet parallel and hips-width apart and rise high on the balls of the feet, pause, and lower the heels
Bridge Lifts	Lying on your back, knees bent, feet flat and hips-width apart, lift butt high, squeeze the butt and lower
Bridge Lifts Single Leg	Same as bridge lifts, except cross right outer shin across the left thigh in a figure-4 shape, push into left foot lift butt squeeze pause and lower
Side-Lying Inner Thigh	Lying on your left side, bend your right knee and right foot flat. Extend the left leg, then lift and lower your left leg as high as your right knee with a flexed foot.
Bicycle Abdominal Move	Hands behind the head, knees into chest, extend the left leg, squeeze the left elbow to the right knee, alternate legs, push low back into the floor

Maintaining fitness for your own well-being does not have to cost a lot or require you to travel. You can get great results with minimal stress right at home!

CONCLUSION

For some, this book may feel overwhelming. To suddenly reincorporate all the self-care habits and best practices that you've let slip over months or even years, that's quite an ask. So let me say it clearly: that is not my intention! **Self-care is a day-by-day process.** With that in mind, my hope is that you'll skim this book often. Some years, one idea may make sense for you to implement; other years, a different idea may take root. I want you to utilize this as a reference to take 5 or use the whole book, whichever is best for you at this moment in time. Get a copy for your best friend or co-worker and go through it together.

I want you to be reminded and inspired to care for yourself. You have already made a serious commitment to be a first responder, essential worker, service man or woman, or caregiver—now it is time to become the best you that you can be, the most productive person at your job, an overall amazing person to be around. This type of living and thinking is what will give you longevity, both on the job and in life. **When we take time for ourselves and take care to spend those 86,400 seconds a day wisely, we can become stronger and more bonded, as humanity is intended to be.**

At its core, caregiving is *giving* and giving is its own greatest reward. We need to remember how it was during the pandemic: how we deeply appreciated the commitment of our essential workers. We valued them so much that we made snacks, donated meals, even rang bells at a certain time of the day to proclaim our gratitude. If you are a caregiver, you can remind others of those times; if you know a caregiver, you can perpetuate a ceremony of your own to keep these essential workers uplifted and motivated to keep going. Caregivers are there for us unconditionally, sometimes at the cost of their own health and the families they love. So before you put this book down, make a list of your own group of caregivers and essential workers in your life and take a moment to send a quick text of love, drop off a meal, offer to take their children for the night, the list goes on. I guarantee your support to other caregivers in your circle will come back to you.

Teachers, childcare workers, agricultural trades, medical services, mental health professionals, critical retail positions, service men and women, transportation professionals: never forget them, always support them and forever care.

APPENDIX:
HEALTH SCREENINGS

I cannot write about self-care and not take a moment to mention the importance of keeping tabs on your health. The following is a list of critical health screenings that individuals should be sure to follow if they want to stay abreast of any changes in their personal health, as well as preserve their health going forward. (Credit goes to the Columbia University Doctors and Nurse Practitioners site.*)

Complete Guide to Annual Health Screenings by Age
Health screenings are an essential aspect of preventative health for people of all ages. Your provider will often recommend tests when you come in.

WHAT TESTS SHOULD YOU GET WHEN YOU ARE FEELING HEALTHY? WHAT TESTS SHOULD YOU ASK FOR?

According to the U.S. Preventive Services Task Force, early detection is critical when treating illnesses like cancer and controlling chronic conditions. There are age-specific tests that may not be needed yearly and specific tests for different genders. Understanding these tests and when to ask for them can help you stay on top of your overall health.

Here is an in-depth guide to the health screenings you might need, organized by age and gender. An established baseline is required for many tests and is often gathered in the earlier years. Each individual may have additional blood work, screenings, and tests recommended by a provider

* www.columbianps.org/healthy-life-blog/guide-to-annual-health-screenings-by-age

based on your personal history. Work with your primary care provider to set up the annual health screenings that are right for you.

18–39 YEARS OLD

Busy work and family lives often keep healthy adults from seeing their primary care provider. Annual health screenings at this age are often missed. A well-person screening is typically covered by insurance and recommended yearly.

This annual screening would typically include the following:

- **Weight and Height:** Annually
- **Blood Pressure:** Annually
- **Cholesterol Check:** Annually, if there are known risk factors; otherwise, every five years.
- **Skin Screening:** For lesions or moles that look suspicious.
- **Historical Illness Screenings:** For known family medical issues such as heart conditions, diabetes, and cancer.
- **Diabetes Screening:** Annually if there are known risk factors; otherwise, bi-annually if BMI is greater than 25 or other lifestyle factors are present.
- **Immunizations**
- **Depression Screening**

Getting blood work done annually is also valuable. These screenings may include the following:

- HDL and LDL cholesterol
- Complete blood count
- Basic or complete metabolic panel
- Thyroid panel
- Liver enzyme markers
- Sexually transmitted disease tests
- Plasma glucose

EXTRA SCREENINGS FOR WOMEN

- **Cervical Cancer Screening**: Pap smears every 3 years.
- **HPV Vaccine**: If not received as an adolescent.
- **Breast Exam**: You should perform a self-exam at home monthly and by a clinical provider yearly.
- **Sexually Transmitted Infections**: Depending on lifestyle or patient request. May include HIV, HPV, Chlamydia, Gonorrhea, or other infections.

EXTRA SCREENINGS FOR MEN

- **Sexually Transmitted Infections:** Depending on lifestyle or patient request.
- **Testicular Exam:** Home self-exams can be done as well.

40–64 YEARS OLD

Based on your medical history, the screenings completed for adults ages 40–64 will continue annually. Work with your provider to determine if these tests can be done bi-annually, every 3 years, or in a different time frame based on current medical issues. Additional health screenings, tests, and vaccines that could be done in this age bracket include:

- **Shingles Vaccine**: Two doses separated by 2 to 6 months given at age 50 and up.
- **Flu Shot**: Annually
- **Colorectal Screening**: Age 50 and up unless other risk factors are present.
- **Colonoscopy**: May be needed based on medical history.
- **Osteoporosis Screening**: Age 50 and up with risk factors.
- **Lung Cancer Screening**: Annually if a past smoker. According to the American Lung Association, adults aged 55 years and up can have this screening covered by their insurance.
- **Depression Screening:** Mental health assessment

EXTRA SCREENINGS FOR WOMEN

- **Annual Blood Work**: Continue annual exams as established in earlier years.
- **Mammogram**: Annually or bi-annually based on your risk factors.
- **Pelvic Exam**: Physical exam and pap smear every 3 years or more frequently based on history and risk factors.

EXTRA SCREENINGS FOR MEN

- **Prostate Exam**: Age 50 and up unless other risk factors are present.

65 YEARS AND OLDER

Many optional tests in the other categories will become recommended by age 65 and are more readily covered by insurance companies. These tests are essential to evaluating overall and maintaining health at this age.

All the previous yearly tests will continue, with these additions:

- **Colorectal Cancer Screening**: Baseline test if not done previously and continued tests based on baseline results.
- **Height and Weight**: Although this is a yearly screening, as you age, height becomes more critical, as shrinking height could be a sign of osteoporosis.
- **Fall Prevention Screening:** Baseline and then as needed.
- **Depression Screening:** Mental health assessment.
- **High-Dose Flu Vaccine**: According to the Centers for Disease Control and Prevention, Fluzone High-Dose is only available to adults 65 and older.

EXTRA SCREENINGS FOR WOMEN

- **Cervical Cancer Screening**: Most women can stop having pap smears if they have no history of cervical cancer. If a hysterectomy occurs, then no pelvic exam may be necessary.

- **Osteoporosis Screening**: Women are at higher risk for osteoporosis and will be screened more regularly at this age. (Baseline at 65 years old, if not already established, and additional screening based on the results.)

EXTRA SCREENINGS FOR MEN

- **Prostate Screenings**: Continue annually.
- **Osteoporosis Screening**: Every 5 years after the baseline is established.

Screenings 101: Your Whole-Body Checklist*

Sometimes, making checkup appointments and blood draws doesn't feel all that important. Health screenings get pushed to the next year or are forgotten entirely. However, getting screenings is one of the most essential things both men and women can do for their health because even being active every day and eating a balanced diet isn't enough to know you are healthy.

Check the lists below to see which screenings (and at what time) you should discuss with your physician so you can be proactive about your health.

- Blood pressure
- Cholesterol
- Type-2 diabetes
- HIV and sexually transmitted infections
- Skin cancer
- Colorectal cancer
- Lung cancer
- Prostate cancer
- Testicular cancer
- Breast cancer
- Cervical cancer
- Regular dental care

* lovelace.com/news/blog/screenings-101-your-whole-body-checklist

MEN AND WOMEN

HIGH BLOOD PRESSURE

Developing high blood pressure is very common, affecting one in three Americans. Get your blood pressure checked every two years if within the normal range and every year if above normal (120/80 and 139/89 respectively).

CHOLESTEROL

The American Heart Association recommends that all adults 20 or older have their cholesterol and other traditional risk factors checked every 4–6 years. After age 40, your healthcare provider will also want to use an equation to calculate your 10-year risk of experiencing cardiovascular disease or stroke, according to the American Heart Association.

Cholesterol testing should also be done at a couple of points during childhood: once between ages 9–11 (before puberty) and once between ages 17–21 (after puberty).

TYPE-2 DIABETES

After age 45, adults should get screened every three years. Screenings should be done earlier if you are overweight, have blood pressure 135/80 and up, have high cholesterol, or have a family history of diabetes. One-third of Americans with diabetes are unaware of their condition, and diagnosing and treating diabetes can have a profoundly positive impact on your health.

HIV AND SEXUALLY TRANSMITTED INFECTIONS (STIS)

Get tested as long as you are sexually active. If you've had unprotected sex, have a new partner, or are worried about infection for any other reason, getting tested is a good idea. Sexually transmitted diseases, including HIV, can be present and show no symptoms. Don't be embarrassed — your physicians want to ensure you are healthy.

SKIN CANCER

Check your skin often for irregularly-shaped, dark spots. Pay close attention to the face, back, and shoulder regions. If you find any concerning marks, make an appointment with a physician. Additionally, have your physician check your skin since it can easily be hard to see your whole body.

COLORECTAL CANCER

Starting at age 45, a fecal blood test can be performed annually. Colonoscopies are performed every 10 years. In 2018, some 140,000 Americans were diagnosed with the disease, and 50,000 died. Experts believe adequate screening could have prevented 60% of those deaths.

LUNG CANCER

Annual screening for lung cancer with a low-dose CT scan in adults ages 55–80 years who have a 30-pack/year smoking history (smoked one pack per day for 30 years, two packs per day for 15 years, etc.) and who currently smoke or have quit within the past 15 years.

MEN

PROSTATE CANCER

It would be best to get screened for prostate cancer at age 55. You should consider getting checked earlier if your brother or father had prostate cancer, if you are African-American, or are experiencing problematic urinary changes.

TESTICULAR CANCER

All men should have a testicular exam as part of their routine physicals starting at age 15. You should also perform self-exams, feeling for hard lumps, smooth bumps, or changes in the size or shape of the testes. Talk to your physician if you have a family history of testicular cancer or an undescended testicle.

WOMEN

BREAST CANCER

Starting at age 50, women should get a mammogram every two years until age 74.

CERVICAL CANCER

A pap test should be performed every three years, starting at age 21 until age 65.

Mental Health Resources

Here is a list of resources from the National Institute of Mental Health. **Call 911** if you or someone you know is in immediate danger, or go to the nearest emergency room.

988 SUICIDE & CRISIS LIFELINE

USE LIFELINE CHAT ON THE WEB (ENGLISH ONLY)

The Lifeline provides 24-hour, confidential support to anyone in suicidal crisis or emotional distress. Call or text 988 to connect with a trained crisis counselor.

VETERANS CRISIS LINE

USE VETERANS CRISIS CHAT ON THE WEB

The Veterans Crisis ChatLine is a free, confidential resource that connects veterans 24 hours a day, 7 days a week, with a trained responder. The service is available to all veterans and those who support them, even if they are not registered with the VA or enrolled in VA healthcare.

DISASTER DISTRESS HELPLINE
CALL OR TEXT 1-800-985-5990

The disaster distress helpline provides immediate crisis counseling for people experiencing emotional distress related to any natural or human-caused disaster. The helpline is free, multilingual, confidential, and available 24 hours a day, 7 days a week.

If you are worried about a friend's social media updates, you can contact the safety teams at the social media company. They will reach out to connect the person with the help they need.

Finding a Health Care Provider or Treatment

Treatment for mental illnesses usually consists of therapy, medication, or a combination. Treatment can be given in person, via phone, or computer (telemental health). Knowing where to start when looking for mental health care can sometimes be challenging, but there are many ways to find a provider who will meet your needs.

Primary Care Provider

Your primary care practitioner can be an essential resource, providing initial mental health screenings and referrals to mental health specialists. If you have an appointment with your primary care provider, consider bringing up your mental health concerns and asking for help.

Federal Resources

Some federal agencies offer resources for identifying healthcare providers and help in finding low-cost health services. These include:

- Substance Abuse and Mental Health Services Administration (SAMHSA): For general information on mental health and to locate treatment services in your area, **call SAMHSA's National Helpline at 1-800-662-HELP (4357)**. SAMHSA also has a Behavioral Health Treatment Services Locator on its website that can be searched by location.

- Health Resources and Services Administration (HRSA): HRSA works to improve access to health care. The HRSA website has information on affordable healthcare, including health centers offering care on a sliding fee scale.

- Centers for Medicare & Medicaid Services (CMS): CMS has information on its website about benefits and eligibility for mental health programs and how to enroll.

- The National Library of Medicine (NLM) MedlinePlus: NLM's website has directories and lists of organizations that can help identify a health practitioner.

NATIONAL AGENCIES AND ADVOCACY AND PROFESSIONAL ORGANIZATIONS

Advocacy and professional organizations can be a good source of information when looking for a mental health professional. They often have information on finding a mental health professional on their website, and some have practitioner locators. Examples include but are not limited to:

- Anxiety and Depression Association of America
- Depression and Bipolar Support Alliance
- Mental Health America
- National Alliance on Mental Illness

State and County Agencies

The website of your state or county government may have information about health services in your area. You may find this information by visiting their websites and searching for the health services department.

Insurance Companies

If you have health insurance, a representative of your insurance company will know which local providers are covered by your insurance plan. The websites of many health insurance companies have searchable databases that allow you to find a participating practitioner in your area.

University, College, or Medical Schools

Your local college, university, or medical school may offer treatment options. To find these, try searching on the website of local university health centers for their psychiatry, psychology, counseling, or social work departments.

Help for Service Members and Their Families

Current and former service members may face different mental health issues than the general public. For resources for both service members and veterans, please visit MentalHealth.gov or the U.S. Department of Veteran Affairs.

Deciding if a Provider is Right for You

Once you find a potential provider, prepare a list of questions to help you decide if they fit you. Examples of questions you might want to ask a potential provider include:

- What experience do you have treating someone with my issue?
- How do you usually treat someone with my issue?
- How long do you expect treatment to last?
- Do you accept my insurance?
- What are your fees?

Treatment works best when you have a good relationship with your mental health professional. If you aren't comfortable or feel like the treatment is not helping, talk with your provider or consider finding a different provider or another type of treatment. Children and adolescents that don't have a mental health professional should consider speaking with a health care provider or another trusted adult.

Only stop current treatment after talking to your health care provider.

NIMH offers basic information on mental disorders and a range of related topics. Printed publications can be ordered for free and are available in English and Spanish. Order online or call 1-866-615-6464.

For all mental health-related questions, requests for copies of publications, and inquiries concerning NIMH research, policies, and priorities, please reach out to the NIMH Information Resource Center using the contact information provided below:

Telephone

1-866-615-6464 (toll-free)

Available in English and Spanish

Monday through Friday

8:30AM–5:00PM ET

Live Online Chat

Live Help

Available in English and Spanish

Monday through Friday

8:30AM–5:00PM ET

Email Us: nimhinfo@nih.gov

Available in English and Spanish

ABOUT THE AUTHOR

GWEN LAWRENCE is a health and well-being educator, mindfulness coach and a practicing fitness professional for over 30 years. Her current work includes specialized self-care and resilience training for healthcare professionals, caregivers, and essential workers. Gwen has been a facilitator,

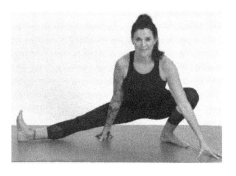

author, speaker, trainer, and yoga instructor. Named "Best Innovation in Sports Medicine" by ESPN Magazine, she is a pioneer in the genre of yoga and sports, training over 3000 professional athletes, and students in 18 countries with her Power Yoga for Sports programs.